Welcome from the Founder of H

Greetings! The fact that you are holding this manual in your hands is evidence that you want to learn the skills necessary to provide a quality, injury-resolving, deep tissue massage. Whether you are a brand new massage therapist or a seasoned professional, this workshop is designed to give you the tools you need to get your clients out of pain....fast!

I have been teaching Secrets of Deep Tissue™ for 14 years to thousands of students. The course content has expanded by over 30% during that time and each technique tested and retested to provide the most effective and long lasting results your client needs. I've used these techniques on my personal clients for the past 20 years with incredibly successful results as well as hundreds of thousands of clients from students, just like you, who have taken this workshop.

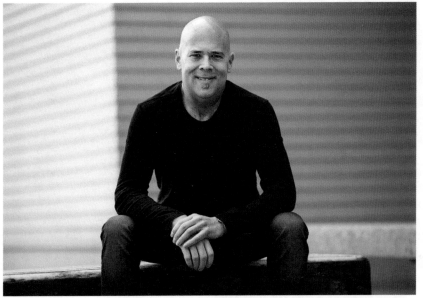

Many practitioners are in search of the "holy grail" of bodywork....the one technique that will truly make them an advanced therapist. In truth, there are only so many ways a body worker can touch and move the skin, fascia, muscles, joints, tendons and ligaments. Techniques are simply the ingredients; the "secret" is in the "recipe" of application of intensity, duration and frequency. It's no different than two chefs using the exact same ingredients yet yielding different results.

I have been teaching Secrets of Deep Tissue™ for over 14-years now and the course grew in content by over 30% in those 14-years. Up until this past year, I also taught a course called Whiplash, TMJD and Intraoral Treatment. Although I teach business courses to help healthcare professionals succeed in making an exceptional and more-than-livable income, Secrets of Deep Tissue™ is the only bodywork course I teach now.

I was personally involved in the early days of Washington State's Intraoral Endorsement law, which would give massage therapists the legal ability to massage inside the mouth if they had additional training and received an endorsement from the state. In the early hearings, there were other health professions attempting to block the law. There were even those who demanded that massage therapists have a 100-hour intraoral training requirement. That's crazy.

The truth is, intraoral massage can be taught in just a few hours and the 16-hour requirement is overkill. It was while I was teaching my TMJD class in 2013 that I had an epiphany: *Since muscular injury affects posture and gait which in turn affect the Temporomandibular Joint, my entire Secrets course was directly related to intraoral training.* At that moment I began the process of merging Secrets of Deep Tissue™ with my TMJD course. With this manual in your hands, I am proud to announce this completely updated and revised 2-day course and I am thrilled that you have decided to join me for an experience that will forever change how you treat your clients and patients.

In Health,

Robert B. Haase, LMP
Haase Myotherapy® Founder

The publisher and author are not responsible as a matter of product liability, negligence or otherwise for any injury resulting from any material or instructions contained herein. This publication contains information relating to general principles of medical massage theory and technique which should not be construed as specific instructions for individual clients or patients.

Technique photos from screen shots of the Secrets of Deep Tissue Technique Video, updated for 2015. Additional technique photos courtesy of Holly Haase, Joseph Lambert and Nadia Joyce Aikins.
Author's portrait by Holly Haase

Models: Kari Taylor, Sara Marie Haase, LMP and Lunden Lisherness, courtesy Heffner Management, Seattle, WA
Illustrations by the Haase Seminars graphics team

Special thanks to our content editors: Charity Lisherness, LMP, Sara Haase, LMP & Lori Logan

©2015, Haase & Associates, Inc.
Updated January 5, 2015

What's Inside...

Notes

Section One: Foundations & Lecture

Haase Myotherapy® Philosophy

- Years in practice vs. consistent, successful results (practicing bad technique doesn't make it correct)
- 20,000+ massages, years of experimentation
- Varicose Vein
- "Dwight"
- Same school, same class, different quality of graduate? Why?
  - Box of ingredients, different result
  - What makes Haase Myotherapy different
  - There is not one technique to fix all injuries
- Autopsy
- Nothing new under the sun… Ecclesiastes 1:9 (New International Version)

  What has been will be again,
  What has been done will be done again;
  There is nothing new under the sun.

  (Written almost 3,000 years ago)

- ALL bodywork techniques fit into just FIVE Categories:
  - Compression – Light & Deep
  - Gliding – Light & Deep
  - Range of Motion – Active, Passive, Resistive
  - Rhythm
  - Energy
- Important changes to thoughts on:
  - Hydrotherapy *ice · 1 min stays cold*
  - The less a muscle is touched the faster it responds to touch
  - Warm-up Theory *don't warm up*
- Tensegrity
- Function of muscles
- Symptoms versus pathology (don't massage the left arm to treat a heart attack)
- Psychology of pain
- Importance of words – Understanding placebo
- Educating your client on the Pain Threshold Theory
- Testing of muscles:
  - Scope of practice
  - False positives
  - Endangerment of patient
- Important to have client show you where it hurts on his/her body and observe *how* they show you

How to Interpret a Client's Description of Pain:

Point: Local
Press: Antagonist
Paint: TP Referral

Perpetuating Factors

- How do you work?
  - Hours, Fatigue
  - Workstation
  - Eye dominance (Go with 1st instinct and do not over-think it)

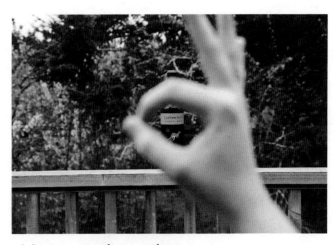

- Activities, repetitive motion
- Duties in relation to posture
- Sit, stand, drive
- Phone use
- Driving
  - Hours in traffic
  - Stick shift vs. automatic
  - Foot well size vs. foot
- "Sleep injuries"
  - Mattress
  - Pillow
  - Position
  - Bolstering
  - Sleep Apnea (4% men, 2% women)
- How do you walk?
  - Footwear
  - Orthotics
  - Leg length
- How do you spend your evenings?
  - How much did you spend in your easy chair?
  - Nighttime nutrition
  - Medications
- General nutrition
  - Water
  - Calcium, magnesium
  - Fish oils
  - Smoking
- Drugs (the "Soup": Anti-inflammatories, muscle relaxants & pain killers)

How did the accident happen?
- When did it happen?
- Did it happen?
- Reality vs. memory
- Trust your hands

Tendon Issues Clarified:
Tendonitis:
 Inflammation of a tendon
Tenosynovitis:
 Inflammation of the tendon sheath
Avulsion:
 Rupture of a tendon

Haase Theory:
Beginnings of Fibromyalgia:
"The Wheel"

- Pain
- Reduced sleep
- Reduced exercise
- Lack of energy
- Instant/prepared foods
- Lack of Hydration
- Toxification of tissues
- Pain

Ending Fibromyalgia:
"Breaking the Spokes"

- Get sleep (even if an Rx is necessary)
- Get exercise
- Whole foods & good nutrition
- Remove allergens (diet and environmental)
- Hyper-hydration
- High-Performance Lymphatic Massage

Tissues & Systems: How They Work & What Can Go Wrong

Mechanical:

- Manipulating Golgi Tendon Organs
  - Manual pressure on muscle fibers allows muscle to relax via GTO's.
  - Caution of vigorous cross-fiber on tendons or muscle will withdraw
  - GTO's need to receive equal stretch on both ends of a muscle to let go (perpendicular stretch)
- The role of a chiropractor
  - Working with a chiropractor
  - Philosophies of treatment
  - Understanding "subluxation"

Nerve Compression...
Only FIVE pounds of pressure for just FIVE minutes on a nerve trunk will diminish transmission by as much as 40%!

- Other spinal/postural considerations:
  - Fascia and posture
  - Bulging/herniated discs
  - Fusions
  - Scoliosis
  - Head Forward Posture correction
  - Extra cervical vertebra
  - Lower Leg Length Inequality
  - Short Upper Arms
  - Small Hemipelvis
- Trigger Points
  - Ischemic Pressure & Stretch

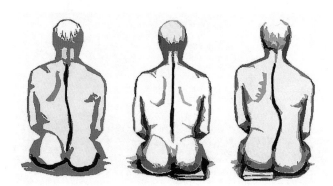

Notes

Massage before chiro adj.
What do you want to do when you are out of this (P)

Section Two: Technique

Golfer's Elbow

Symptoms: Client will usually show signs of pain, tenderness, stiffness, weakness, numbness and tingling.

Golfer's Elbow = Medial Epicondylitis (inflammation of the medial epicondyle and surrounding tissues.) Usually from repetitive use.

Golf swing often cause/origin of pain, in addition to chopping wood with an ax, chain saw work and hand tool use.

Most of the wrist flexors join together and attach to ONE main tendon, the Common Flexor Tendon, attaching to the medial epicondyle of the humerus. Overuse puts strain on this tendon causing inflammation and/or scar tissue.

Standing in front of your client, have her extend her left upper arm toward you with the forearm towards the ceiling at a 90° angle (flexed), internally rotated and hand relaxed. As you face her, hold her left hand/wrist with your right hand and press your left thumb into the painful area of the forearm below medial/superior end of the Ulna. Press firmly with direction toward the Olecranon Process (tip of the elbow.) Acute conditions will require firm cross-fiber friction for 30-seconds. (Ice the area following the sequence if cross-fiber is performed.)

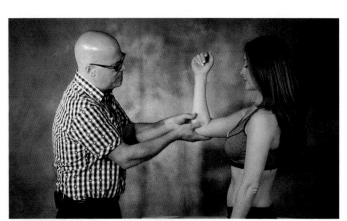

While maintaining pressure with your thumb, open the arm by extending and rotating the forearm until the upper and lower arm are completely straight and extended. Release your pressure and then return the forearm to its flexed, internally rotated position and start again.

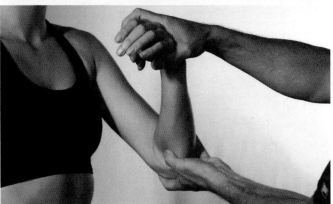

Acute conditions will need you to add 30-seconds of aggressive cross-fiber friction on the tender tissues, followed with 30-60 seconds of ice massage or wrapping the wrist in an ice pack. Ice until the skin remains cold to the touch for a full minute after icing. Be careful not to burn the skin with ice.

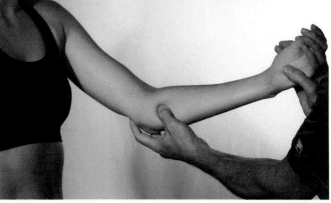

Symptoms: Client will usually show signs of pain, tenderness, stiffness, weakness, numbness and tingling.

Tennis Elbow = Lateral Epicondylitis (inflammation of the lateral epicondyle and surrounding tissues.) Often as a result of repetitive use.

In tennis, a backhand swing can cause the problem, as does painting with brush or roller, chain saw work and repetitive hand tool work. Note that grasping can worsen the condition.

Symptom: Pain at the lateral epicondyle, spreading down forearm. Some clients can not fully extend (straighten) the arm. Note that Radial Tunnel Syndrome is often mistaken for Tennis Elbow, but if in doubt, the massage treatment is the same.

Standing to your client's left side with her arm in front of you as the upper arm is abducted, forearm flexed with palm to the floor. Use your right hand to grip and press your fingertips into the muscularity surrounding the lateral epicondyle, directing force towards the Olecranon Process (tip of the elbow.) Acute conditions will need you to add 30-seconds of aggressive cross-fiber friction on the tender tissues, followed with 30-60 seconds of ice massage or wrapping the wrist in an ice pack. Be sure not to burn the skin with ice and ice until the skin remains cold to the touch for a full minute after icing.

With a smooth motion, maintain pressure on the tender tissues with your fingertips as you extend the forearm. Try the same motion while adding a turn of the client's hand into a supine position.

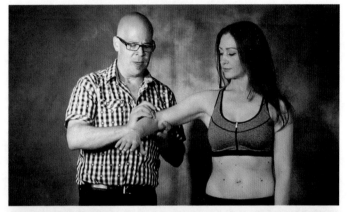

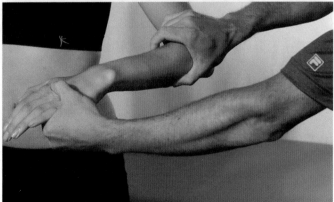

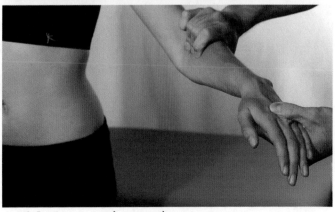

Carpal Tunnel Treatment Sequence

Symptoms: Pain, numbness and tingling in the area of the arm that is supplied by the median nerve. Pain may radiate proximally. Can have numbness/tingling of palmar surface of any of fingers, except the little finger. Additional symptoms with degree of severity.

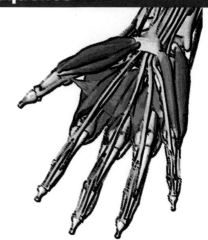

Median nerve passes through tight tunnel, surrounded by carpal bones, filled with ten tendons of the fingers and thumb, strapped-in by transverse ligament.

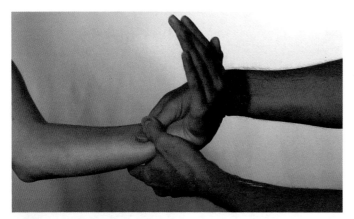

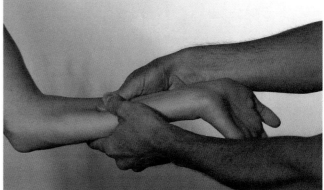

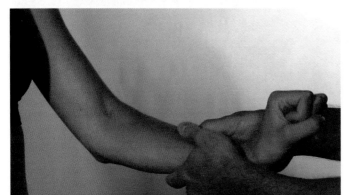

Above: Pin & Stretch Flexors, Passive: Use "shortened muscle" techniques by holding her fingers as straight as possible while you pin & stretch with depth and a fairly brisk rhythm along the flexors (anterior forearm.)

Active: Perform same motions with reinforced thumbs, one thumb over the other.

Left: Pin & Stretch Extensors, Passive: Continue on the extensors (posterior forearm) while you have your client make a fist to enhance the stretch. These areas may be tender, so work within your client's tolerance.

Active: Perform the same motions with reinforced thumbs, one thumb over the other.

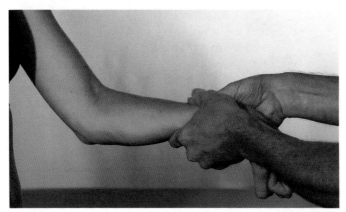

X-Fiber/Grind: With pressure, work cross-fiber on the Transverse Carpal Ligament and Flexor Retinaculum (about an inch or so above and below the "wrinkles of the wrist") in all directions.

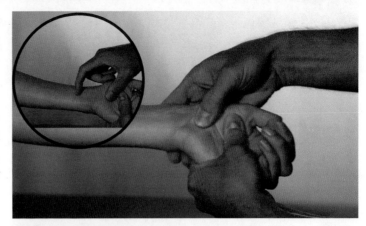

Work with firm and specific intent to break up adhesions and bring nutrition to the structures. You will want to work aggressively with your thumbs, as though you are trying to rub off a temporary tattoo.

"Rock & Roll": By firmly grasping the carpals with your hands and rocking them back and forth you can help increase ROM in the joint.

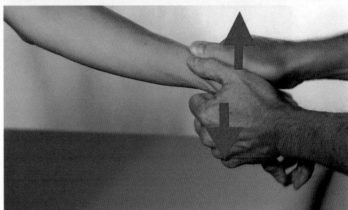

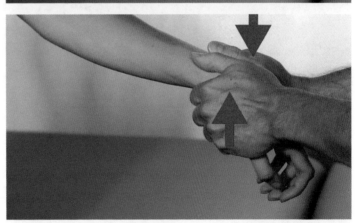

Follow the "rock" with a "roll" over the joint. Simply pinch the carpal bones together and then make a small, firm, smooth "wave" with the bones, allowing them to work through their range of motion. It is a "Squish and Spread" movement. All you are looking for is movement/mobility in the joint.

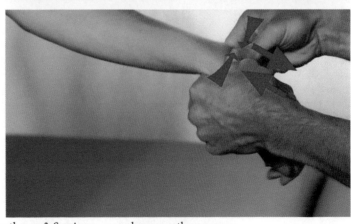

CAUTION: ALWAYS perform ice massage or wrap the wrist following aggressive treatment on your carpal tunnel clients.

Symptoms: de Quervain's Tenosynovitis/ Tendonitis creates painful inflammation of the thumb's tendons on the lateral (thumb side) of the wrist. Pain with turning the wrist, grasping, gripping or making a fist. Rare instances of an audible "chirp" can be heard.

De Quervain's Disease involves painful inflammation of the two tendons in the thumb that extend the wrist, the Extensor Pollicis Brevis and Abductor Pollicis Longus muscles. The swollen tendons and their coverings friction against the common sheath that they share.

In this photo, the client is performing the Finkelstein maneuver which is used to diagnose de Quervain's Tenosynovitis. If a client feels pain, during ulnar-deviation, when she grasps her thumb with her fingers while making a fist, most likely she has de Quervain's. If the client only feels discomfort in this area during the Finkelstein test, she will be able to benefit by beginning the healing process prior to a potential acute phase.

Using one hand to mobilize her fist, use your other hand to work the tendons and tendon sheaths of the Abductor Pollicis Longus & Extensor Pollicis Longus muscles with your fingertips and thumbs.

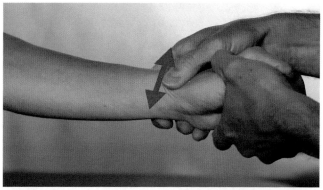

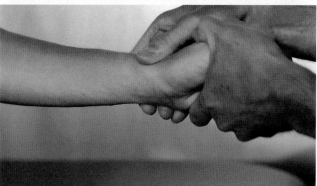

Bring the fist into radial-deviation, apply pressure with your thumb or fingertips, then move the fist into ulnar-deviation, and then release the pressure. This will be uncomfortable. You will most certainly need to apply ice after the technique. In acute stages you may find that applying ice prior to the technique will provide an analgesic effect, reducing any discomfort your client may experience. Repeat the pin & stretch technique several times, followed by ice massage.

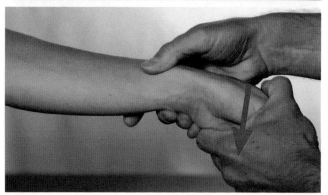

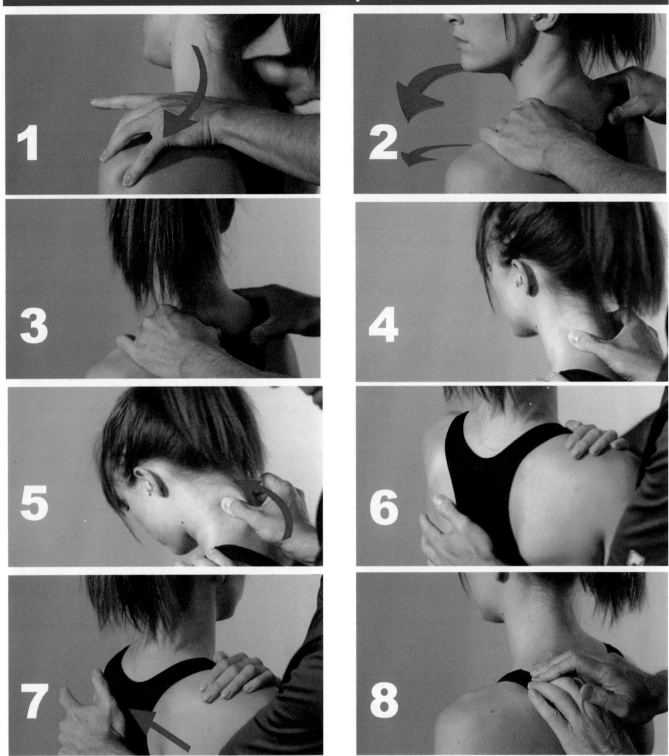

1: Firmly compress the upper trapezius while guiding your client's head into lateral neck flexion with a "palm-glide" down the trapezius , 2-3: With "duck-billed" fingers, pinch the upper trapezius, have the client laterally rotate head, opposite direction, 4-5: Using one hand to pinch the posterior cervicals, have the client flex her neck anteriorly. Release the pressure, actively or passively bring the head back to an upright position and repeat. 6-7: Standing to the client's left side, have the client place her right hand onto her left shoulder. With your left hand, grasp her right elbow and

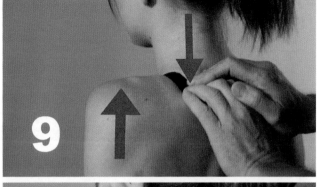

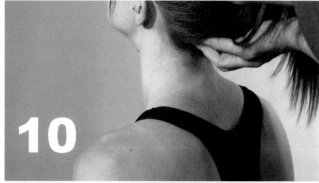

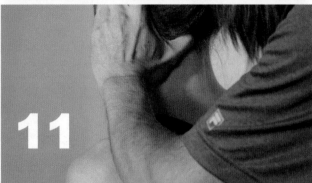

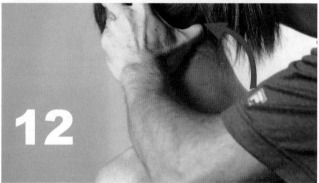

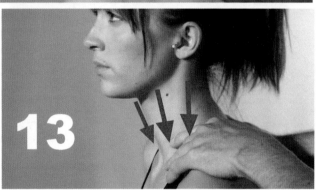

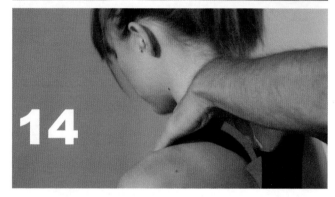

rotate her torso in a counter-clockwise direction while you use your thumb, fingers or heel of your hand to glide from the medial border of her right rhomboid and glide to the lateral border on the medial scapulae border. Return her to the starting position and repeat, 8-9: After frictioning the insertion of the Levator Scapula, use Active/Resistive technique by resisting your client's attempt to elevate her shoulder while you apply pressure to the levator scapula insertion, allowing full range of motion under resistance. 10: Let your client's head drop back into your cupped hand, massaging the occiput with circular tips on suboccipitals. 11-12: Follow with gentle pin & stretch on the suboccipitals using thumb compression, extension to flexion. 13-16: Using a combination of flat fingertips and reinforced thumbs, work around your client's neck systematically with pin & stretch movements. Work all cervical muscle groups with extra caution around the scalenes. Work around entire neck, 360°. Continued on next page...

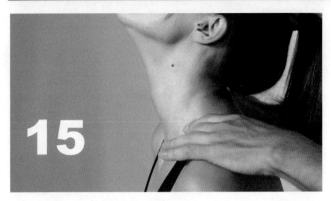 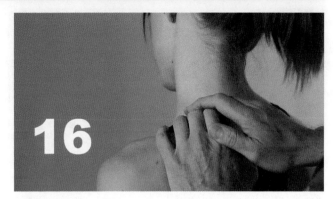

15-16: Continue "360-degree" pin & stretch work around the neck.

Notes

If it hurts, rub it

Rectus Abdominis Treatment Sequence

Symptoms: Rectus Abdominis is involved in maintaining postural distortion that usually originates from shortened "hamstrings". Once shortened hamstrings are addressed, the Rectus Abdominis must be lengthened to allow for erect posture to resume. Note that trigger point pain referral patterns from a Rectus Abdominis TP can mimic acute appendicitis (photos, right.) Once appendicitis has been ruled out, treat the referred pain patterns with this technique sequence.

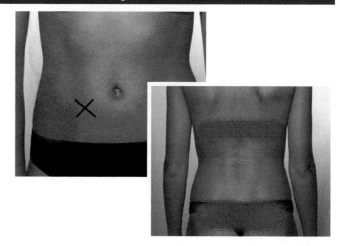

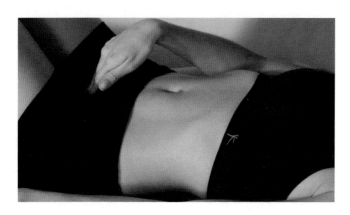

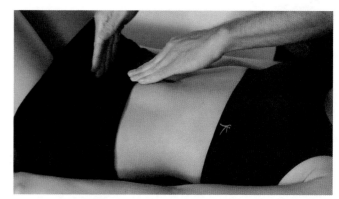

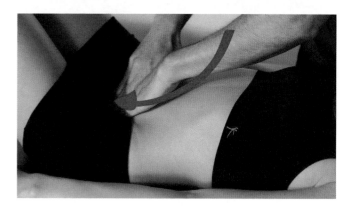

Have your client lay on her back, supine, with her feet flat on the table, knees up. Explain the procedure in detail and obtain permission. Have her place one hand on her pubic bone and keep it there. This will provide her with a safety barrier for her and let you know your relevant landmarks. Overlap your fingertips to about the 2nd knuckle while making an obtuse angle. Place hands flat on lower abdomen approximately 2-3 inches superior to her pubic bone.

Have client take a deep breath. As she exhales, drop down and under the pubic bone and hold firmly as she exhales and hold firmly as she inhales against your resistance. Release your pressure before the exhale and allow her an unrestricted breath, and then repeat several times. You can also try using your two thumbs, about 3-4 inches a part, at the lower Rectus Abdominis.

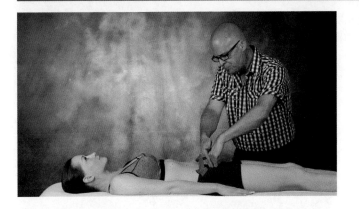

With cupped fingertips (reinforced if necessary) hover with vertical palm angle and cross-fiber the insertion of the rectus abdominus at the pubic bone. Work firmly and be sure to keep the palm as vertical as possible while still maintaining firm pressure.

Remember, do NOT hover over their genitals. Rather, keep fingers in a more vertical position.

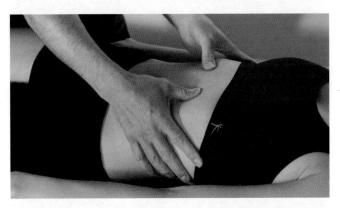

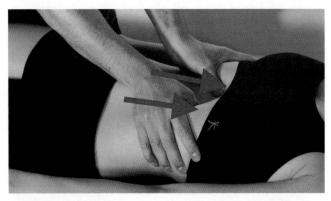

To stretch the upper fibers of Rectus Abdominis, place your thumbs about 2-3 inches below the lower ribs. As your client takes a deep breath, follow the exhale with your thumbs, swinging up and under the lower ribs with a vertical path. Hold the pressure as your client creates a stretch with her deep breaths against your resistive pressure.

As you stretch the Rectus fibers under the rib cartilage, being careful of the Xiphoid process. Maintain a distance of an inch or so between your thumbs as you straddle the Xiphoid.

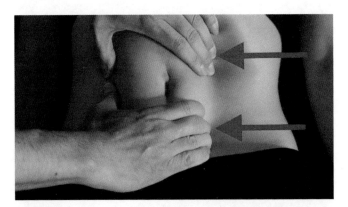

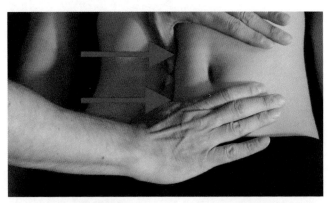

To release the trigger points, particularly the trigger point that resides in the lower right lateral quadrant (the one that refers pain mimicking acute appendicitis), stand at your client's side. Use horizontal thumbs to push the border of Rectus Abdominus away from you, holding for 5-10 seconds. Then pull

the far border of the muscle using your fingertips to "rake" towards yourself, holding for 5-10 seconds. Repeat for several times for a total treatment time of 2-3 minutes. If the referred pain subsides, the sequence is complete.

Adductor Treatment Sequence

Symptoms: Adductor spasm and general tension-based issues result in pain and decreased range of motion. Gate will usually be affected resulting in postural compensation.

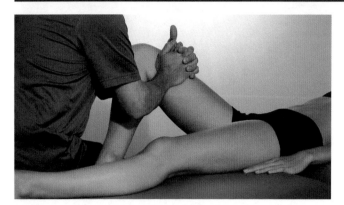

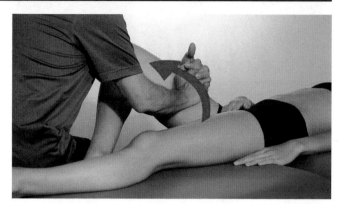

With your client lying supine, bend one knee and place the foot of that leg flat on the table, against the medial aspect of the other knee, as shown above. Interlocking your fingers, make your arms into a "hoop" around her leg. Bring her knee fully upright and use the heel of your inside hand to apply pressure to the adductors and press firmly as you drop

the leg into external rotation. Do not twist the bellies of the muscles. Release the pressure, bring the leg back to a vertical position, reposition the heel of your hand and repeat. Work your way down the adductors until you reach the inguinal triangle. Be sure to use your client's hand as a boundary at the pubic area.

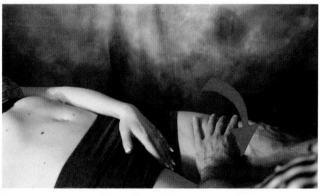

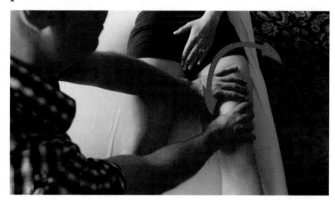

Standing across the table, have your client internally rotate her leg into your resisting thumbs. Work

all of the adductors. Use her hand as a protective boundary.

Notes

Symptoms: Sciatica and "false sciatica" both have radiating pain from the low back, through the buttock and down both legs. Piriformis impingement of the sciatic nerve ("false sciatica") can be differentiated from actual sciatica by relief from muscle treatment and home stretches. Keep in mind it takes several days to observe nerve impingement relief.

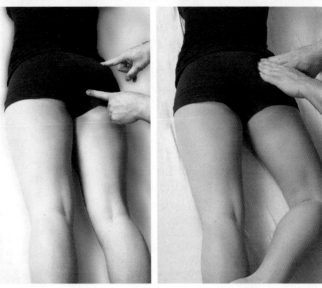

When a client has sciatica-type symptoms, be sure to assess if the piriformis muscle may be involved. More often than not, the piriformis muscle is pinching the sciatic nerve rather than an impingement of the nerve by a herniated disk of the lumbar spine. Treatment: Place the leg as shown by bringing the knee out to the client's side into external rotation. Their foot will rest at their calf muscle or at the back of the knee of the other leg. Isolate the origin of the piriformis at the sacrum by pressing against the lateral border with your fingertips. Then follow the edge of the sacrum to the iliac crest and mark with one finger as you also follow the edge of the sacrum down to the coccyx bone and mark with another finger. The piriformis will be exactly 1/3 the distance from your two fingers marking both ends.

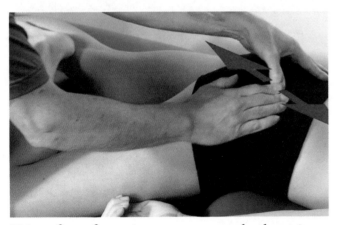

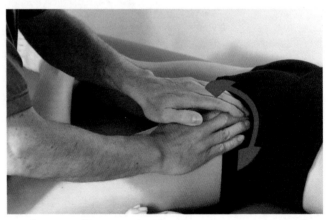

Using firm fingertip pressure, work the trigger points with static/ischemic pressure as well as with vibration at the sacral attachment. You should also work cross-fiber on the piriformis origin as well as the insertion at the greater trochanter.

Notes

Standing to your client's side while she is in a prone position, hold the lower leg in an upright position by the ankle with the hand closest to the foot. Externally rotate the leg by lifting the lower leg vertically and pushing the foot away from you. With the other hand, make a tight fist and place your knuckles with pressure against the piriformis at the lateral border of the sacrum (you may also use your flat forearm.) While holding pressure on the muscular attachments at the sacrum's edge, pull the foot toward yourself so that you internally rotate the leg. Once the leg reaches its end-feel, release your fist pressure and repeat.

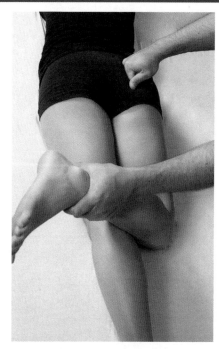
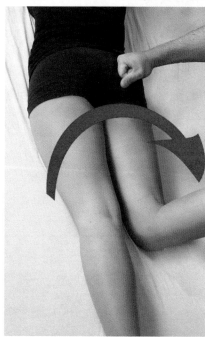

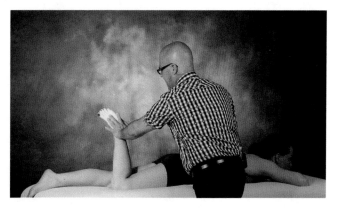
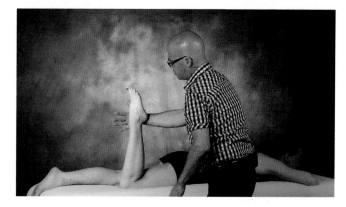

Finish sequence with PNF work. Support ankle as the client internally and externally rotates leg against resistance using "2-push, 2-pull" technique.

Notes

Symptoms: Gluteus Medius and Minimus lay one on top of the other, with the Minimus being the deeper. Originating below the Iliac Crest and inserting on the Greater Trochanter, these muscles work together to abduct the hip as well as offer both internal/external rotation and flexion/extension of the hip. Gluteus Medius problems are often the result of Morton's Toe/Morton's Foot Structure. If Morton's Toe is present, a podiatrist can fit a quality orthotic to compensate for the problem. Morton's Toe not only leads to problems with the Gluteus Medius, but eventually will affect the Vastus Medialis and Peroneus muscles. Fatigue and trigger point referral patterns are common, as shown to the right.

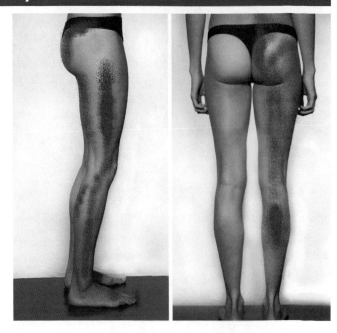

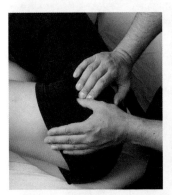 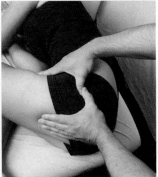

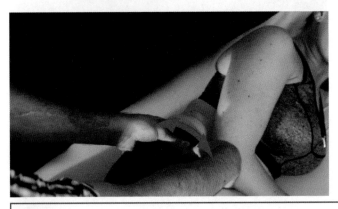

Treatment: (Photos, Left) Position client on her side, with buttocks at the very end of the table. Client holds her knees to her chest. Work the Gluteus Medius and Minimus muscle bellies, just below the Iliac Crest. Force is downward (use your palm to press your thumb bone into the muscles. Also use reinforced thumbs up under the illiac crest with cross-fiber friction as well as around the attachment on the Greater Trochanter of the Femur.

Using reinforced thumbs (laterally positioned, thumb over thumb), work up and under the Iliac Crest at the most lateral aspect. Being mindful of the intensity of the discomfort that this technique can cause, work firmly and slowly, cross-fiber on the most superior origins of the Gluteus Medius and Minimus muscles.

Notes

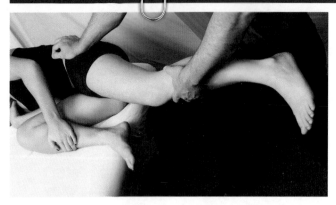 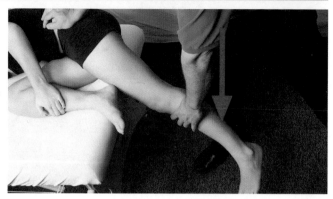

Standing to the back of your client, support her lower leg with your hand that is closest to her foot while you extend her upper leg. Have her continue to hold her other leg to her chest. Lift her leg to an elevated position and then use the heel of your upper hand to apply pressure on the bellies of the Gluteus Medi-

us and Minimus. As you maintain pressure, lower the leg to create a "pin-and-stretch" effect. Repeat several times with the leg at various degrees of flexion and extension. You may find that utilizing your elbow, parallel to the floor, is easier on your body.

Knee & Upper Leg Sequence

Symptoms: Regarding the I.T. Band, some clients go beyond a "stuck" or tight Iliotibial Band and have a condition called Iliotibial Band Syndrome which can be identified by symptoms ranging from stinging just above and lateral to the knee to swelling and/or thickening of the band along its length. It can also appear just below the knee at its insertion.

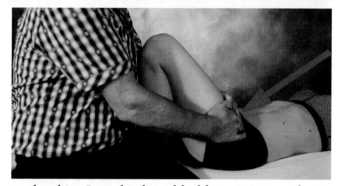

Sitting on the table, place your client's foot under your thigh. Use your looped arms to hold pressure at the very top of the thigh applying direct contact

to the skin. Lean back and hold tension in order to decompress the hip. Hold tension for 10-15 seconds and repeat 2-3 times.

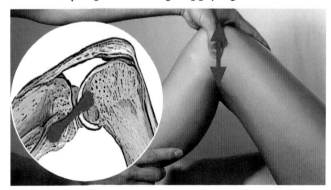 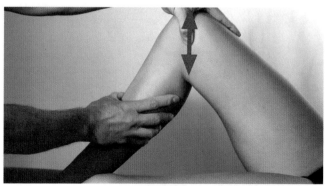

With knee at a 90° angle, find the groove between the fibular head and the medial femoral condyle. Similar to two fists bumping into each other, the lateral and medial collateral ligaments serve as straps on both sides of the knee to hold the mechanism to-

gether. Simply use your thumb to rub the ligament, cross-fiber, between the two bones. If the ligament is the issue, it will be exquisitely tender to the touch. After 30-seconds of vigorous cross-fiber friction, follow with 30-60 seconds of ice massage.

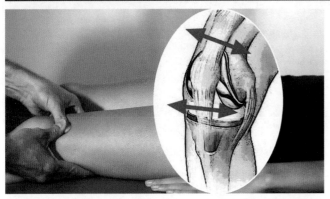

Using reinforced thumbs, work cross-fiber both immediately above and immediately below the patella.

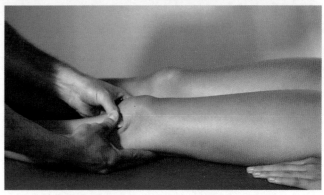

Work firmly and with constant speed, approximately 1/2 to 1-second from side to side.

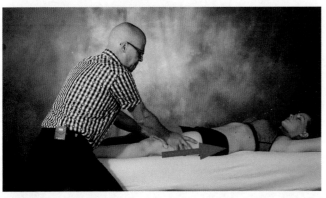

Similar to the I.T. Band fascial tug, use the palm of your hand to stretch the fascia of the upper leg on the inside, top and outside aspects. You may also

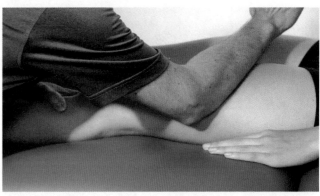

want to use the belly of your forearm as a tool to work with pressure, relieving your wrists of stress.

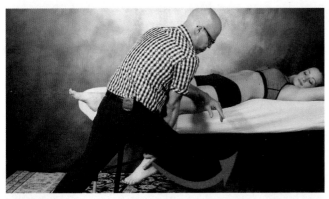

Abducting the leg off of the edge of the table, use your forearm to apply deep, even pressure, while flexing the knee as you draw the lower leg up and

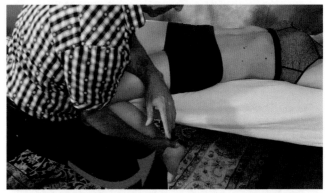

under the table. This is a specific pin & stretch movement. Repeat up and down the bellies of the quadriceps group.

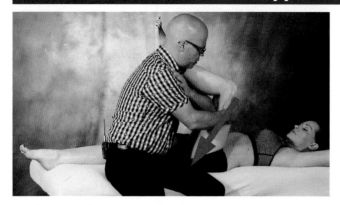

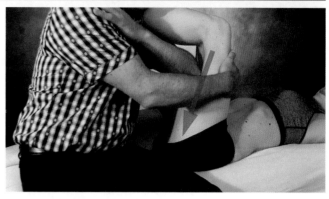

With your client in a supine position, lift their leg as shown in the above left photo and use your elbow to strip down between the bellies of the Biceps Femoris. You can also use your straight-wrist-fist as you deeply glide (slowly and very little oil) from

behind the knee to their Ischial Tuberosity. Try lifting the foot slowly for a glide & stretch. You can also perform Hybrid PNF on their straight leg from this position.

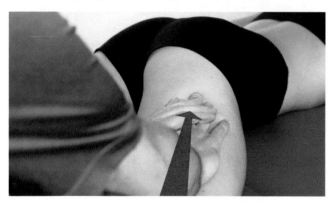

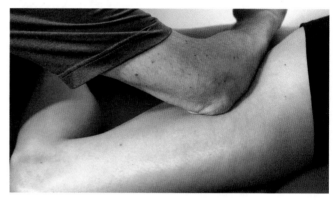

With your client prone, place her upper leg into the "frog leg" position (externally rotated, knee flexed.) Without lubricants, place one palm over the other

and use firm pressure to drag from the knee to the greater trochanter. Use "fascial speed." You might also use your forearm to save your hands.

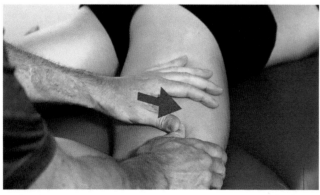

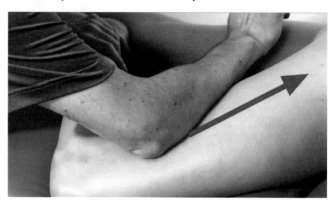

Use reinforced thumbs (one over the other) to slowly and firmly "strum" over the IT Band, broadening the fibers while working within your client's pain tolerance. An optional myofascial release would be to use your forearm belly to tug up the IT Band with

firm pressure and no lubricant, use myofascial intent/pressure/speed to stretch up the I.T. Band fibers. Pressure should be controlled, slow and in the direction of the hip.

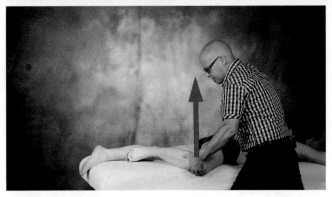

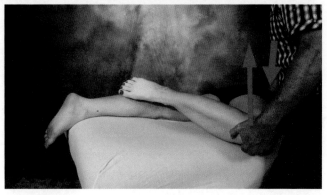

With your client's leg in the "frog leg" position, use your palm to press down on the sacrum, holding the low back down to the table. With your other hand, slowly and firmly lift the knee up towards the ceiling. DO NOT lift more than 1-INCH. This stretch is subtle yet powerful. Not everyone will feel the stretch, but those clients who need the stretch will definitely feel the movement. Please stay in communication with your client during this stretch.

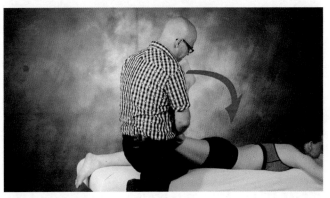

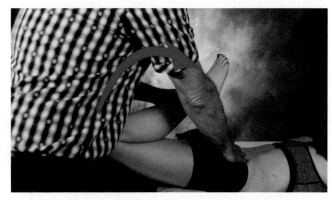

With your client prone, lift her foot off of the table, place your knee on the table and then rest her knee on top of yours, placing her quads into a gentle stretch. Gently enhance the stretch as you push down on her ankle, moving her foot towards her buttocks, flexing the knee and maximizing the stretch. As this stretch is quite effective, go slow and stay in constant communication with your client.

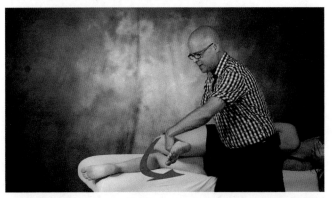

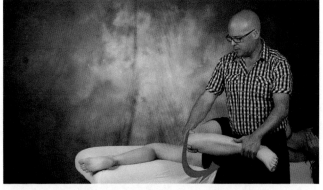

With your client side-lying next to the edge of the table, support her knee and ankle, keeping her leg level with the floor. Press your hip into her low back, almost facing away from her. Slowly bring her leg around you while keeping constant pressure into her low back and her hips perpendicular to the table. Slowly draw her leg around you and hold the stretch. Repeat 2-3 times.

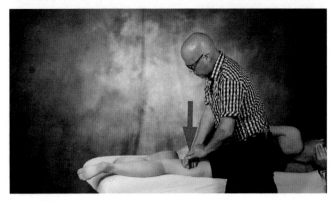

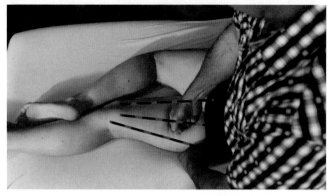

As your client is side-lying with her bottom leg extended and upper hip flexed, press your fists downward into your client's adductors, quads and hamstrings, working along the three lines shown. When

working the hamstring line, press downward and then roll slightly backwards. Press every couple of inches for 2-seconds each.

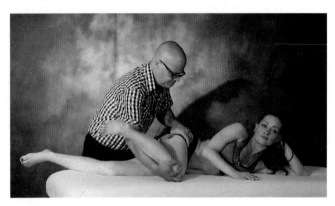

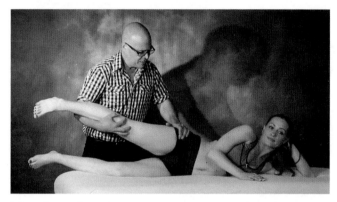

To stretch out trigger points and spasm in the Tensor Fasciae Latae (TFL), start with client side-lying towards the side of the table. Use your arm to cradle and support the knee and lower leg as shown. Let the knee drop to the table as you internally rotate her leg, essentially lifting the lower leg off of the ta-

ble. Place firm fingertip pressure on the TFL, gripping it as you lift the knee and straighten the leg so that it is parallel with the table. In short: Knee starts down towards the table with foot raised, pressure is applied to the TFL, then leg then straightens. Release the pressure and repeat.

You can perform this technique using both of your hands while reinforcing your fingers. The client will make the movement actively with your verbal instruction. (Shown in photo, left.)

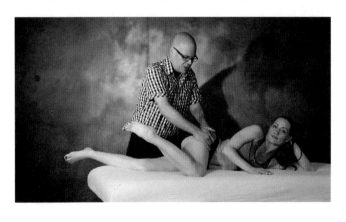

Sacrum & Pubic Symphysis Release

Symptoms: When the Sacrum and/or SI Joint (sacrum/Ilium) experiences dysfunction, the client typically experiences pain that is aggravated by sitting, bending over and standing. Severe issues can refer pain into the hip, leg and groin areas. Occasionally you may encounter a client that has previously fallen on their "tail bone"/Coccyx that resulted in the Coccyx bone pointing directly anterior. This can be addressed by a chiropractor in some states throughout the USA.

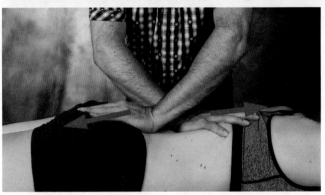

Placing one hand on your client's sacrum and another on her low back, use firm pressure (without lubricant) to spread the fascia and decompress the sacrum and low back.

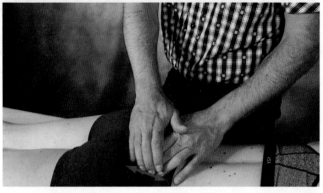

Work the entire lateral borders of the sacrum with cross-fiber friction. Use either reinforced fingers as you reach across the table or thumb-over-thumb on the border closest to you.

Using your hand to reach across the superior lateral borders of the sacrum, as you drop over each side, your fingers and thumb drop into the SI joint and SI ligament, running head to toe (generally.) Cross-fiber friction for 30-seconds to 1-minute.

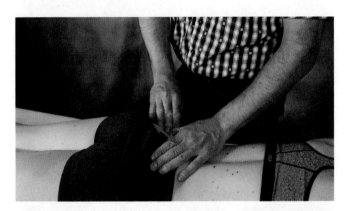

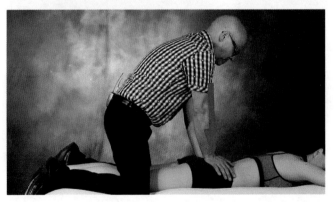

With your client remaining in a prone position, kneel on the table, hovering over her knees as you put direct downward pressure on both SI joints. Your fingers should be facing outward and your pressure is applied with the heels of your hands. Keep your arms vertical so that the pressure is downward toward the table.

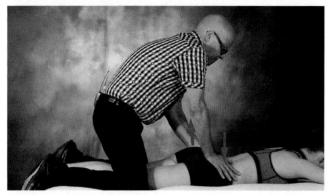

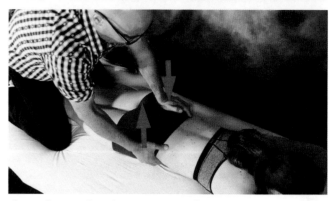

Begin alternately lifting the ASIS (anterior superior iliac spine/front of hip bone) of one side of the pelvis while simultaneously pressing down SI joint on the other side, then reverse the movement, lifting the other ASIS as you press the opposite SI joint. Repeat for 12-sets.

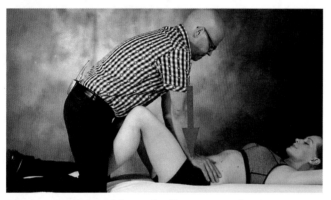

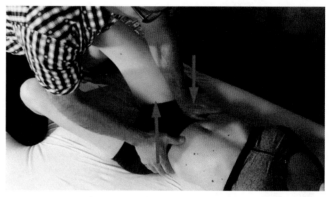

Dismount the table and allow your client to reposition into a supine position with her knees bent, knees slightly apart. Repeat the steps above, but from the supine position. Start with downward pressure on the ASIS bones, holding for a minute or so. Then, begin alternately pressing down on one ASIS while lifting the pelvis by reaching under the hip with flat fingers.

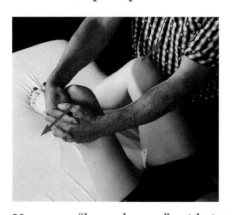

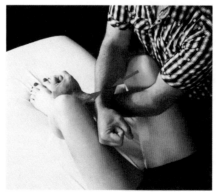

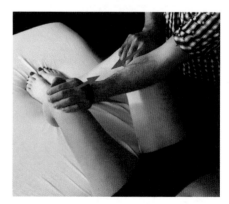

Use your "looped arms" with interlocked fingers as your client presses her knees outward/laterally with isometric pressure as you resist her movement. Perform for 15-seconds or so up to 3-sets. Now, reverse the movement by having her bring her knees together as you resist the pressure. Use either the cross-armed brace (above center) or fix your arms and hands (above right) to inhibit movement. 3-sets of 15-second isometric compressions. The duration and number of sets are a suggestion only.

Bicipital Tendonitis

Symptoms: Bicipital tendonitis is what I refer to as the "fifth shoulder muscle" because it radiates pain in the shoulder, especially when the client lays down to go to sleep at night. Flexion of the elbow against resistance can be painful. It can also be tender to resist supination while the elbow is flexed and the arm is in adduction. It always hurts with direct palpation (cross-fiber) on the tendon or musculotendinous junction.

Bicipital tendonitis is what I refer to as the "fifth shoulder muscle" because it radiates pain in the shoulder, especially when the client lays down to go to sleep at night. Flexion of the elbow against resistance can be painful. It can also be tender to resist supination while the elbow is flexed and the arm is in adduction. It always hurts with direct palpation (cross-fiber) on the tendon or musculotendinous junction.

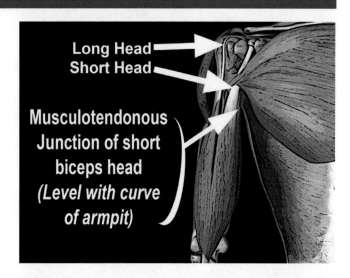

Long Head
Short Head

Musculotendonous
Junction of short
biceps head
*(Level with curve
of armpit)*

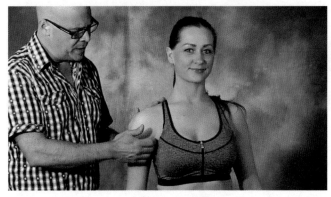

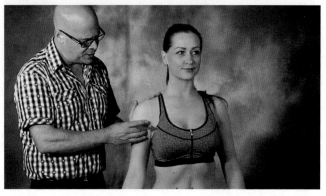

With thumb, straight or bent fingers, friction the medial head of the bicipital tendon, working cross-fiber. Work with firm pressure for at least 30 seconds, but no more than 1 minute. This technique will be uncomfortable to the client.

Follow the treatment with ice massage in a "with-fi-

ber" direction. Ice formed in small paper cups seems to work best. Be sure to use paper towels to instantly wipe any stray ice water as the ice melts. Increased inflammation will cause the ice to melt more quickly. Ice should be used for approximately 30 seconds, or until the area remains cold after icing.

Notes

Symptoms: Supraspinatus tendonitis usually exhibits pain at the outer lip of the AC joint when the client abducts the arm or raises it overhead.

One of the four shoulder girdle muscles, the Supraspinatus muscle is responsible for elevating the arm and moving it away from the body the first 15 to 20 degrees.

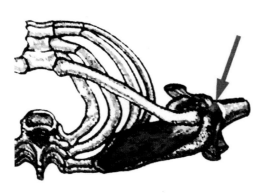
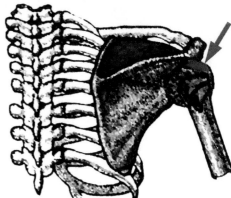

The Supraspinatus tendon is protected by the AC Joint which hovers above. When the client places her arm behind her back, however, the tendon will come out from hiding, enabling you to perform cross-fiber friction.

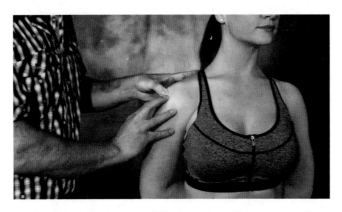
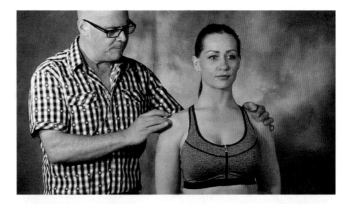

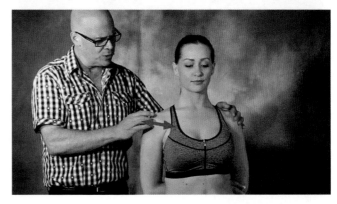

With your client seated facing away from you, place her arm behind her low back and hold it gently in place with your knee. If you choose not to use your knee to passively hold the arm, have your client hold it in place with her opposite arm. Locate the most lateral aspect of the Acromion Process at the shoulder. As you put your finger on the bony edge (above), drop over the lip and follow the ridge about 1-inch anteriorly. At that point you will feel a vertical band which is the Supraspinatus Tendon. If it is the issue, it will be very tender.

Work with cross-fiber friction with as much intensity as your client will allow (no more than a 7 or 8 out of 10.) Work the tendon for 30 to 60 seconds and follow-up with an ice cube or ice cup for the same duration.

Low Back/Psoas Release

Symptoms: Low back pain is fairly self-explanatory. Although there are many potential causes, this treatment protocol has proven effective in relieving pain immediately, regardless of the pain's origin simply by decompressing the structures that are involved. Note: When addressing low back pain, it is usually most effective to begin by releasing the Quadratus Lumborum before releasing the Psoas. Also, if your client presents with pain in her right low back, you will most often find that she will have a significant level of spasm in her left Psoas muscle. This is a component of structural balance. Begin treating the Quadratus Lumborum that is in the least amount of pain.

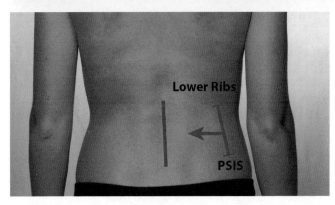

Lower Ribs

PSIS

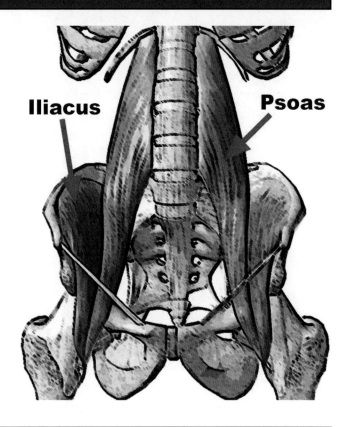

Iliacus

Psoas

To locate the point to apply pressure on the Quadratus Lumborum, find the midpoint between the lowest floating ribs and the top of the Iliac Crest (See above.) Palpate the spinous processes at that mid point, follow across the lamina groove, then push your horizontal thumbs up against the lateral belly of the Quadratus Lumborum which is directly beneath the Erector Spinae. Your pressure should be under the lip of the muscle and downward at a 45° angle.

Notes

after 2-3 hrs of being (P) free after Tx - chiro needed site after next (m) session

2-3 day - just a (m)

do (LB)/psoas last in Tx

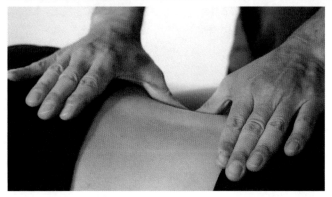 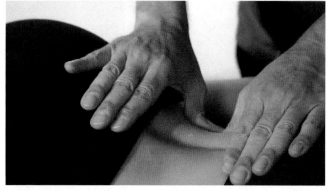

Now that you have located the Quadratus Lumborum, apply pressure with horizontal thumbs while the client gently moves her low back into flexion and extension… this desensitizes the area a small amount. If there is any sharp pain on movement, discontinue movement and perform static pressure work only.

With pressure perpendicular to the lumbar vertebrae, work with downward pressure at a 45-degree angle. Be careful not to go too far laterally as to mistakenly put pressure on the transverse processes of the lumbar vertebrae. Hold static pressure for TP work first. Then have your client perform a posterior/anterior pelvic tilt (flexion/extension) at the pelvis and low back. Photos above show flexion on the left and extension on the right.

In order to save your thumbs from overuse, you may find it easier to utilize the point of your elbow (olecranon process) to hook up and under the Quadratus Lumborum. Be sure to keep your forearm firmly in place with your upper arm coming down into the QL at a 45° angle while your forearm is completely vertical (90°) and your wrist remains relaxed.

With each flexion and extension, regardless of whether you are using your thumbs or elbow, allow the client to lift and lower your elbow/thumbs, up and down. The pressure down and forward (45° angle) remains constant, but the vertical movement is

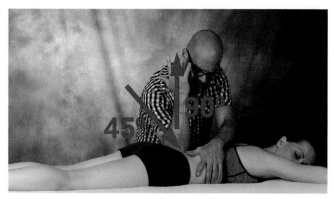

elastic, moving up and down with each flexion and extension.

Notes

heel cup
ice bottle for Plantar Fasc. do it just before bed. don't walk on feet for ½ hr after icing

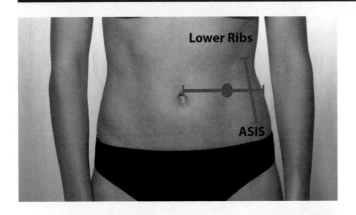

Lower Ribs

ASIS

To locate the point to apply pressure on the Psoas portion of the Iliopsoas muscle, locate the halfway point between the lowest floating ribs and the ASIS. Then find the halfway point between the Linea Alba (vertical mid-line of the abdomen) and the lateral edge of the abdomen. Find the intersection of these two halfway points.

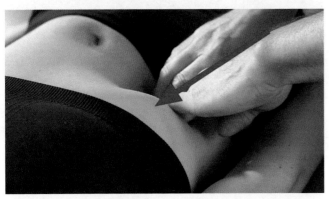

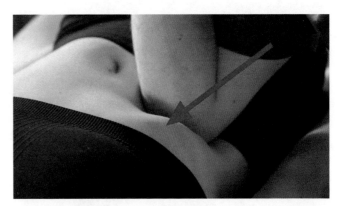

With your client laying supine with bent knees, place your broad overlapped fingertips at the intersection of these four landmarks in preparation of dropping into the abdomen at a 45° angle, pinning the Psoas muscle against the "backboard" of the lumbar spine, pinning the Psoas Major & Minor against the sides of the vertebral bodies. Remember to drop in slowly and incrementally.

As the client breathes normally, gently drop in with each exhalation, and then pull out as she inhales. Your depth will slightly increase with each exhalation. After several breaths, you will be able to palpate the Psoas and literally be pressing against it. Even if you cannot feel the muscle belly, following the previous steps will place your hands right on the outer edge of it.

On the third exhalation, pin the muscle down against the spine and hold it firmly as your client takes a *slow*, deep, 4-6 second abdominal breath. Press harder as she breathes in so that her breath

does not allow your hands to be pushed out. Release the pressure before your client exhales, give her a "free resting breath" and then repeat for a total of six breaths. I find it enhances the release if the client holds the last breath for an extra 4-5 seconds after the full inhalation.

Have your client get off the table immediately with your assistance. Have them get up slowly and hold her arm to stabilize her. If she is undressed, have her use the sheet for a "toga" wrap for purposes of modesty.

Watch for the aortic pulse on the client's left side. In rare occasions you may feel the pulse on the right side. Simply pull back and drop below the aortic pulse. You may also use your elbow so the client is more comfortable with the sensation of pressure. It also helps to use your elbow if the pressure is uncomfortable for your fingers or feels too sharp to the client.

Suggested Low Back Pain Relief Self-Stretches
Twice-Daily or as Directed by Physician

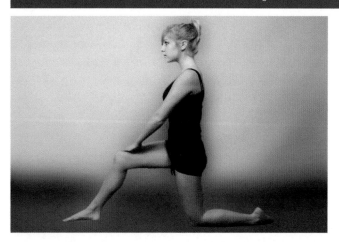 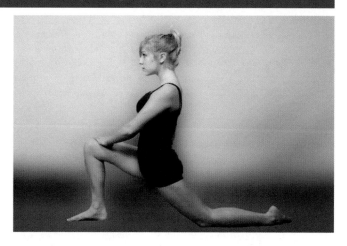

When the client is out of the acute phase of low back pain and injury (low back pain is no longer extremely painful and no longer feels "unstable"), the Iliopsoas stretch is quite beneficial. Have the client start by positioning herself while resting on one

knee while the other leg is extended with her foot out in front of her at approximately a 120° angle, as shown above. She should gently rock forward and hold the stretch 5-8 seconds. Repeat several times on each side.

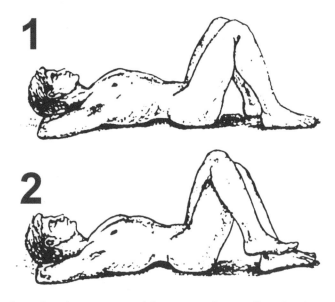

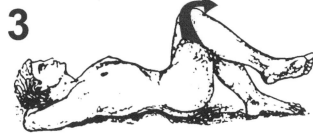

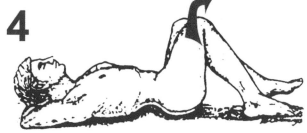

When the client is out of the acute phase of low back pain and injury, the Quadratus Lumborum stretch can bring significant relief from low back pain and can help prevent it as well.

Have your client lie on his back, knees bent and feet

on the floor. Bringing the left leg over the right (#2, above), have him drop both knees/legs to his left side and pause for 5-8 seconds. He will feel a stretch in the low back. If their is sharp pain, he should stop the stretch immediately. Have him repeat the stretch several times on each side.

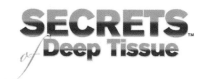

©2015 Haase & Associates, Inc., Haase Myotherapy® Seminars - www.haasemyotherapy.com

Symptoms: Shin Splints will present with a variety of symptoms, usually including pain along the tibia which can run from superficial to deep. Intensity of pain depends on your client's specific case.

The tibialis anterior, with a large and weak connection to the anterior tibia, finds itself being pulled away from the bone, resulting in "shin splints." To treat, we want to increase circulation with ischemic pressure as well as lengthen the muscle, allowing it to have reduced tension during the healing process.

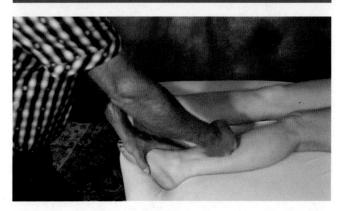

With your client laying supine as you stand at the foot of the table, hold her foot with your inside hand to assist in keeping the leg internally rotated. Using your tightly-closed fist, make sure that you keep your wrist straight and fist out in front of you as you glide. Stay on top of the muscle and away from the

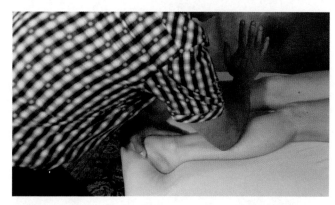

lateral borders so that you do not accidentally press into the Tibea bone. Press down on and glide along the Tibialis Anterior muscle from ankle to the knee. Work slowly and slightly deeper with each pass. You might also try using the flat of your forearm bone (ulna) for deeper work.

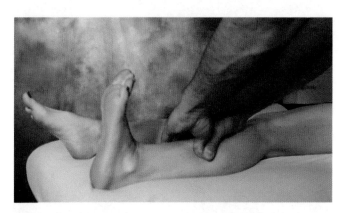

Have your client put their foot into plantarflexion and press your reinforced thumbs into the distal aspect of the Tibialis Anterior muscle belly. This is an active movement. While holding pressure, have the client move her foot into full dorsiflextion and then return it to full plantarflexion. While she momen-

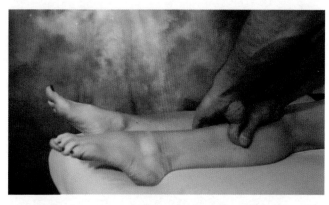

tarily pauses her movement, release the pressure and move your thumb pressure about ½" proximally up the muscle belly and again press into the muscle. Have her repeat the full dorsiflextion and plantarflexion and repeat the process until you reach the head of the Fibula.

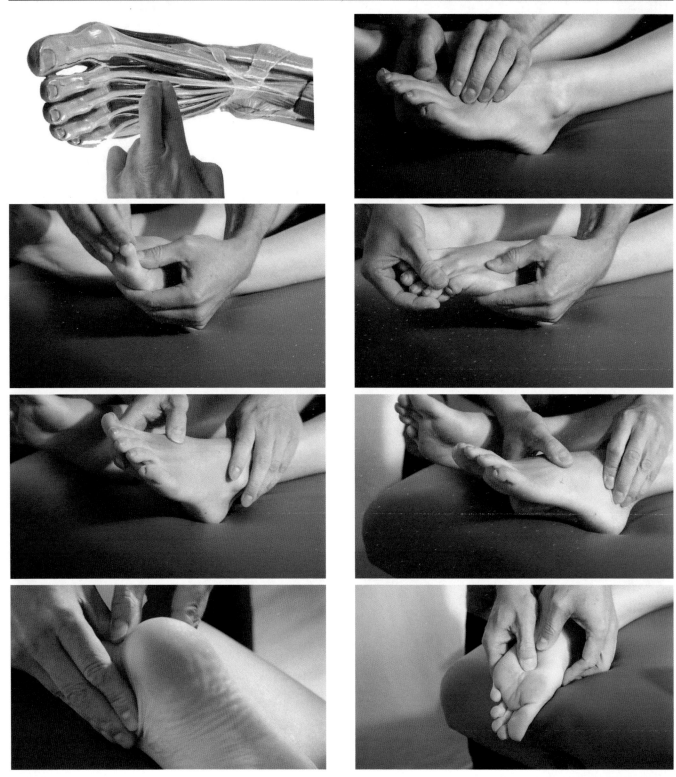

With your client supine, use your fingertips and edge of thumb to work between the tendons of the foot. Using pin & stretch and pin & glide, work the tendons of each toe through its full range of motion. Work the entire ankle around the heel and Malle-olus with friction strokes. With your client prone, continue working the entire ankle with reinforced and gliding thumbs, working the entire plantar surface of the foot.

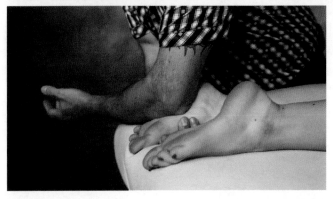

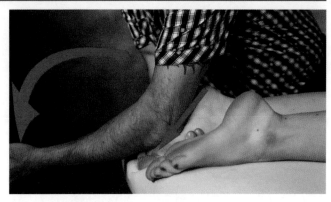

With your client prone, stand facing the foot of the table with your hip touching the side of the table. Use your outside hand to support the foot while the inside arm rests perpendicular to the foot and elbow just below the heel. Glide down the foot as

you simultaneously swing your forearm until it is parallel with the foot. Glide from the anterior edge of the Calcaneus bone until you hit the base of the phalanges (start of the toes.)

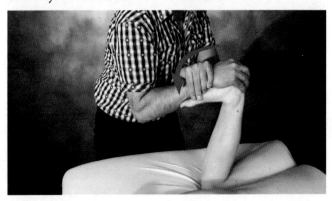

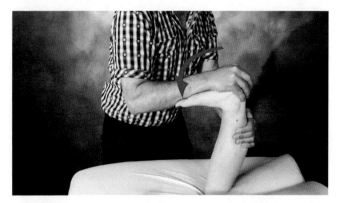

To stretch the calf muscles, place the palm of one hand over the client's heel while your forearm rests on the plantar surface of the foot. You can use your other hand to press down on your own forearm to

stabilize as you press down. Performing a pin & stretch by pinching the calf works well in this position.

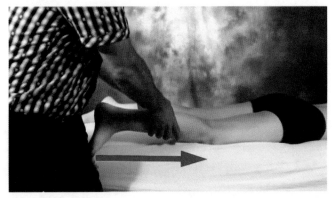

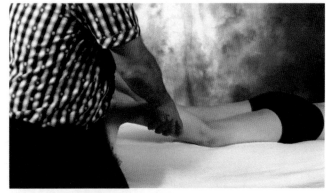

To enhance the stretch of the calf muscles, bring the client's foot off of the table edge, place it on your ASIS, pinch her calf muscles and lunge forward for the stretch. Be sure to either step back enough so

that her heel does not come to rest on your body or turn her foot enough so that it misses your torso entirely.

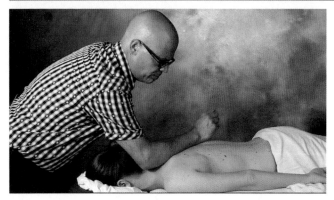

Standing at the head of the table, use your forearm without lubricants to work from the upper Trapezius fibers, down the Erector Spinae, and over the Rhomboids. Work with a deep gripping "tug" of the

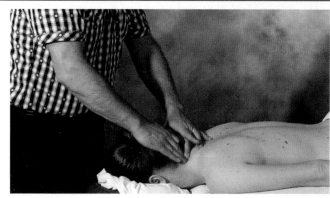

tissues, holding, slowly stretching the tissues as you patiently wait for a slow myofascial stretch. Follow with specific work of the posterior cervical muscles using reinforced fingertips and/or thumbs.

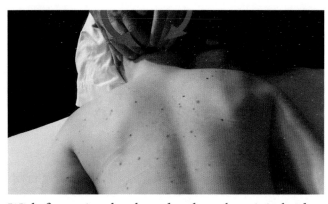

With fingertips, hook under the suboccipital ridge, working the muscles and muscular attachments. Seek out both spasms and trigger points, holding pressure for 4-7 seconds at each TP. Follow by using

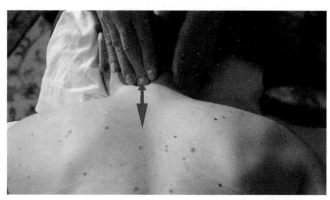

your fingertips or the edge of your thumbs to work in the lamina groove, making sure to work specifically and slowly from head to toe throughout the neck area. Work with deep, specific pressure.

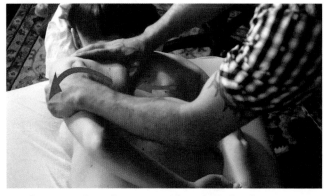

With your client's arm on her low back, use your lower arm to reach across the table and cradle her upper arm from the middle of the Humerus. Lift the arm off of the table and pull it towards yourself. As you allow the arm and shoulder to fall back to the table, use your thumb or the heel of your upper

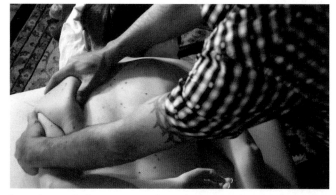

hand to glide out on the Rhomboid muscles. The entire arm and shoulder girdle will lower to the table as your thumb or heel of hand simultaneously glide laterally. Repeat several times. Do not use this technique if your client has elongated rhomboids ("winged scapula".)

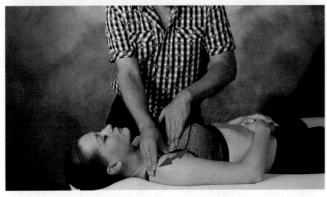

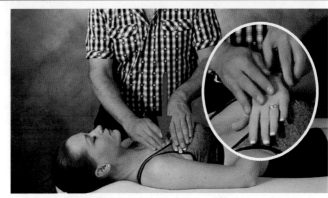

Work the Pectoralis Minor with "local pin & stretch" techniques, working the superficial and deeper fascial tissues, pulling the tissues in opposite directions under moderate to deep slow-moving pressure.

You will likely want to use the client's own hand as a boundary (above right inset.) Continue working the Pectoralis Minor muscle belly with deep trigger point pressure.

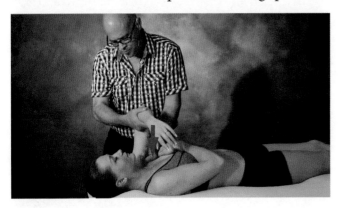

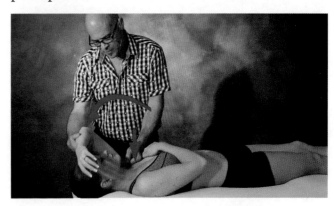

Standing at the client's side, lift her upper arm vertically, bending the upper arm as it hovers directly over her neck and use your hand to support her arm next to her elbow. So that you do not end up giving your client stretch marks with this stretch, it is important that you alleviate the superficial tissue tension before stretching the muscle itself. To do this, you will want to us your lower hand to make a fist, then press it down slightly into her superficial tissues near the breast. Then drag those tissues an inch or two upwards to where you will apply pressure on the pectoralis minor. As you firmly press straight down onto her pectoralis minor muscle, bring her arm up and over her head, her arm brushing along her ear. The movement is similar to a martial arts block with her

upper arm moving in a straight line upwards with no lateral movement. Release the pressure on the muscle and repeat several times. You might also want to use your flat Ulna of the forearm to apply pressure as it is smoother than the bones in your fist (below, right.)

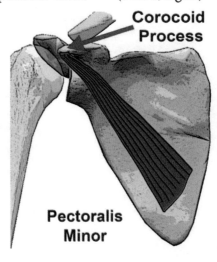

Corocoid Process

Pectoralis Minor

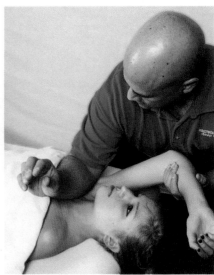

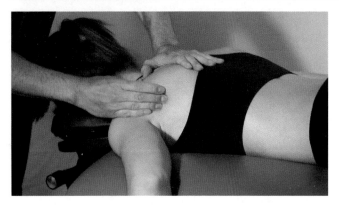

Work the trigger points along the lateral border of the scapula, pressing every 1/2 inch or so.

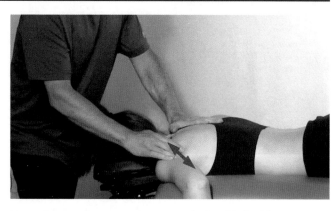

Just above the armpit toward the Deltoid, you can palpate the Infraspinatus tendon. Press down on it until you locate the tendon, then proceed with cross-fiber friction, followed by ice if indicated.

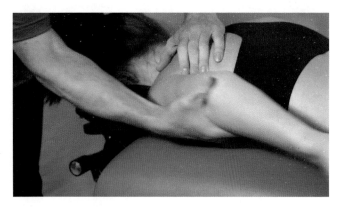

Returning to the trigger points along the lateral border of the scapula. After releasing the trigger points, stand at the head of the table. Continue compressing the trigger points and hold while you abduct the

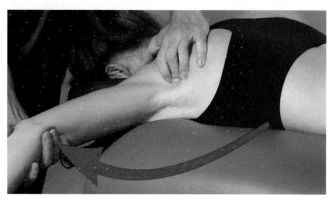

arm. Release the pressure and repeat several times per side. You can do the same with the Infraspinatus tendon as well.

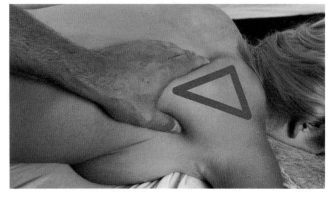

Infraspinatus, one of the four muscles holding the arm in the socket, is best treated with simple trigger point work. Simply outline the inferior borders of the scapulae and the spine of the scapulae. Then

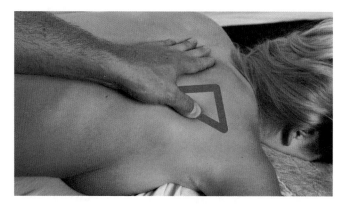

reduce the areas by one inch, creating a smaller triangle. Treat with trigger point work - you cannot miss. The more severe the trigger point, the farther the referred pain pattern will travel.

Subscapularis/Frozen Shoulder Treatment

Symptoms: "Frozen Shoulder", often referred to as Adhesive Capsulitis, results in stiffness, pain and limited range of motion in the shoulder. Most clients suffering Frozen shoulder literally have their arms stuck to the sides of their torsos.

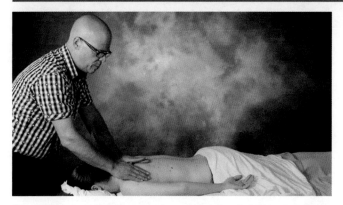

The Haase Myotherapy™ method of Subscapularis treatment is with the client prone. The reason we do this is so that the client is less likely to want to assist and hold her arm up for you as she might in a supine position, engaging the very muscle we are attempting to treat. Stand at the head of the table with your client prone. It is important that and her arms rest on the table along her side.

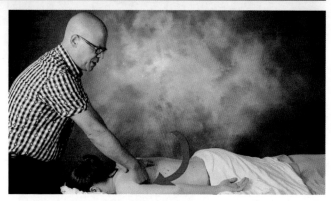

Use an "excessive" amount of oil or lotion to smooth the entire Axilla/armpit. Smooth in circular movements until the entire surfaces are lubricated, allowing uninhibited movement of your fingers.

As your outside hand slides along the side of your client's ribcage, drag your fingertips along the table-top and then up and into the axilla.

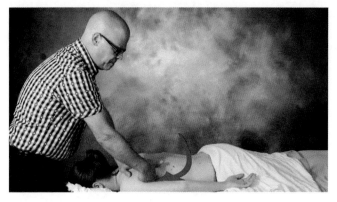

Flex/curl your fingers into a locked position and press up against the Subscapularis while pressing down onto the Scapula with the other hand. Press any trigger points firmly for 5-10 seconds each. For distraction, try using circular movements with the hands working in tandem or use a vibration to relax the muscle.

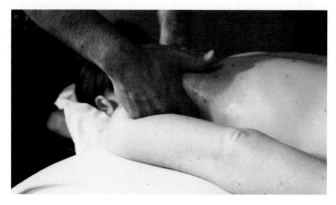

Be careful to stay along the posterior Axillary wall and against the Subscapularis muscle belly itself. Ask your client to tell you if she feels any tingling sensations. If so, back off the pressure and move ½" or so and try again.

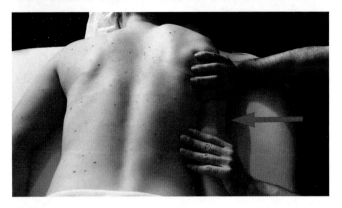 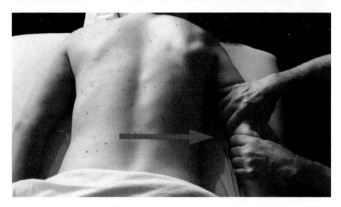

When treating frozen shoulder/Subscapularis, what is not immediately released by direct compression work is nearly always released by the "hybrid" combination of PNF/MET Active Stretches. This technique will offer immediate increased functionality. To utilize the "Hybrid" combination of PNF/MET Active Stretches, begin by supporting the upper and lower arm, starting at full adduction. Have the client take a deep breath while pushing against your pressure (abduction) with 20-25% (or so) of her strength for approximately 3-5 seconds. You will be resisting her pressure so that her pressure is isometric, or without movement. Have her release the active abduction and her breath simultaneously. Bring the arm out a few inches and repeat.

The third time, reverse your support and have her actively attempt to adduct her arm while you resist her pressure. Again, she is using 25%, or so, of her strength while holding her breath, for approximately 3-5 seconds. Move her arm another inch or so and repeat.

The idea is to continue an isometric resistance to her pressure, while she holds her breath, in series of two each: Two isometric abductions, followed by two adduction attempts. Keep repeating the cycles until you reach normal range of motion, or until she has no strength to resist you. Treating "Frozen Shoulder" with this technique is often very uncomfortable for the client to receive. Keep in mind that although extreme discomfort is normal when treating frozen shoulder, sharp pain in the shoulder capsule is not. If there is sharp pain, discontinue the treatment and refer her back to her physician for further evaluation before reattempting the technique.

Notes

Foundations of Temporomandibular Joint Disorder Treatment

What is "TMJ"? Do you have it? If you have a mandible, then you probably have a temporomandibular joint. The question is, do you have TMJD, or temporomandibular joint dysfunction (disorder)? TMJD is a generic term that encompasses acute or chronic inflammation or degradation of the temporomandibular joint, which connects the mandible to the skull, or cranium. The human jaw can exert 200 pounds of force on the molars.

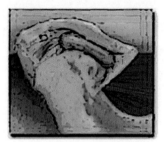 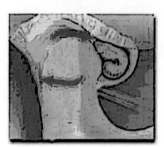 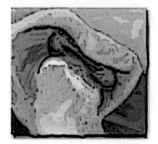

Normal Disc   Disc Displacement   Degenerative Joint Disease

TMJD:

- Can affect one side or both sides of the TM joints
- Can affect the client's ability to speak, chew, eat, swallow, make facial expressions, and even breathe
- Client's may experience other symptoms and medical conditions as a part of a broader multi-system illness, such as:
  - Allergies
  - Headaches
  - Fibromyalgia
  - Sleep disorders
  - Tinnitus

Diagnosis will often be confirmed from a combination of the following symptoms:

- Pain is the most common symptom. TMJ pain is often described as a dull aching pain in the jaw joint and nearby areas, including the ear, which comes and goes.
- Misdiagnosis can lead to "let's try this" treatments, such as a root canal
- Some people, however, report no pain, but still have problems using their jaws, such as:
- Being unable to open the mouth comfortably
- Clicking, popping or grating sounds in the jaw joint

- Locking of the jaw when attempting to open the mouth
- Headaches
- A bite that feels uncomfortable or "off"
- Neck, shoulder and back pain
- Swelling on the side of the face
- Ringing in the ears
- Ear pain
- Decreased hearing
- Dizziness
- Vision problems

TMJD Notes

- Often from malocclusion
- Most TMJD patients are women (95%)
- Why? Common thought is stifled emotions or inability to communicate stress or anger, resulting in clenching of the jaw
- Patient should be able to place 2-3 finger knuckles of dominant hand in their bite (45-60mm)

How TMJD Can Get its Start

- Injuries to the jaw area
- Pterygoid TP's activated with SCM issues
- Digastric TP's from SCM issues
- Increased pain/spasm decreases jaw ROM
- Various forms of Arthritis
- Dental procedures
- Genetics
- Hormones
- Low-level infections
- Auto-immune diseases
- Stretching of the jaw when inserting a breathing tube before surgery
- Clenching or grinding of the teeth (Bruxism)
- Leg length differences (LLLI = Lower Leg Length Inequality)
- Medial Pterygoid trigger points can cause head-forward posture, putting stress on mandible
- Front of Zygomatic arch should be directly above manubrium of sternum
- Anterior deviation of posterior cervical neck should be about 6cm on average adult:v

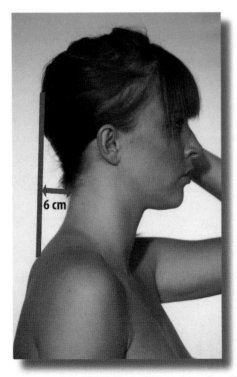

Common Treatments

- Eating soft foods
- Applying ice or moist heat
- Avoiding extreme jaw movements (wide yawning, chewing gum)
- Medication
- Vitamin/mineral supplements
- Botox injections
- Stretching exercises
- Stabilization splint (bite plate, night guard)

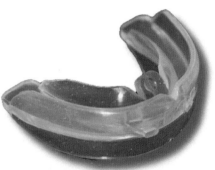

- Manual adjustment via grinding the teeth
- Crown or bridge work to reposition/balance bite
- Surgery:
  - TMJ Arthrocentesis: It involves inserting needles inside of the affected joint and washing out the joint with sterile fluids. On some occasions, the procedure can also include inserting a blunt instrument inside of the joint. The instrument is used in a sweeping motion to remove tissue adhesion bands and to dislodge a disc that is stuck in front of the condyle (ball) inside of the joint.
  - Open TMJ Surgery: Displaced discs can be repositioned and sutured in a more posterior position, among other repairs
  - TMJ Arthroscopy (incisions made and micro-tools are used):
  - Replacement of TMJ or Discs
  - Can increase pain, cause permanent damage or break

Perpetuating Factors

- Excessive head-forward posture
- Chronic mouth breathing
- Acute overload (gum chewing, etc.)
- Nail biting
- Jaw clenching
- Bruxism
- Childhood thumb sucking

Indications for Treatment

- Patients with pain originating from the muscles of the face, head or neck
- Patients with pain in the muscles related to mastication
- Patients with muscle spasms or muscle tension related to TMJD symptoms
- Patients with headaches related to muscle tension

Contraindications

- Active oral lesion (e.g. herpes)
- Abscess
- Intraoral infection
- Neoplasm (tumor or tissue containing growth)
- Contagious infectious conditions of the skin of the face, head or neck including Thrush, Strep Throat, etc.
- Hypermobility of jaw
- Don't make it looser!

Cautions

- Be aware of traumatic instabilities in the TMJ
- Is there joint damage from the injury?

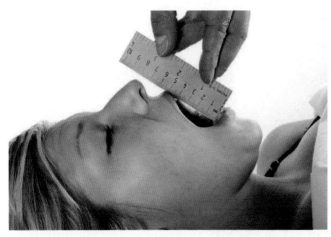

Be sure to measure your client's range of motion in millimeters before and after treatment. Use a disposable paper ruler or a ruler that can be sterilized.

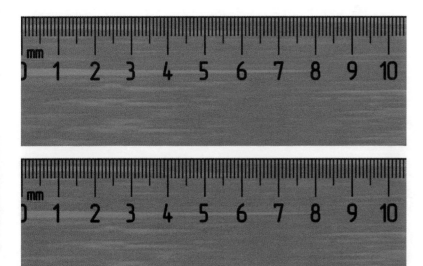

Copyright release is given to photocopy these rulers to the left. Make sure you copy at "100%" (do not "reduce to fit" or enlarge, ensuring accurate ruler measuring. Simply use scissors to trim and keep in a safe and clean location, free from potential contaminants.

Measurements should be made inside the client's mouth opening, measuring the space between the upper and lower teeth.

> *Treat every client as though the client has a contagious disease. Therapists should consider some or all of the following precautions to protect themselves, as well as the client.*

Mandatory

- Health history MUST be taken on any client, prior to treatment.
- What is the client's chief complaint?
- What is the history of the client's chief complaint?
- Has the client ever experienced "locking" of her jaw?
- Does the client have any infection present, or a history of infection?
- Is there a history of any unusual pain in the head, neck or jaw?
- Wash hands prior to treatment
- Note: Hands should be washed with warm, soapy water, before and after each treatment, regardless of glove usage.
- Soap should be dispensed via a pump-type dispenser, not a bar of soap.
- Lathering and rinsing 3-times in a 30-second period is better than lathering and rinsing once in a 3-minute period.
- Purpose of the soap is to break down the surface tension and dissolve oils on the skin

Equipment Notes

- Hand washing station should ideally be nearby the client treatment area.
- Towel dispensers should be hands-free automatic, "C", bi or multi-fold type.
- Chart notes should be done without gloves. Pens should be clean.
- Face masks should be considered to reduce the possibility of fluid splatter being passed to or from the client's mouth.
- Eye protection, such as goggles, safety glasses or a face shield should be used to reduce the possibility of fluid splatter being passed from the client to the therapist.

Gloves:

- Use disposable/single-use gloves. Latex, if client does not have a latex allergy. Gloves MUST be properly disposed of after use on each client.
- Gloves should be stored in an easily accessible, clean area.
- Once gloved, hands should not touch any unclean surface.
- Any cuts, scrapes or wounds on the therapist should be covered (e.g. with a finger cot) Bandages do not work since they will get moist beneath the glove.

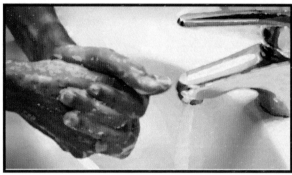

- No jewelry may be worn beneath the glove. You cannot clean around or beneath a ring or bracelet and it could tear the glove.
- De-glove without touching contaminated surfaces with your bare hands.
- The therapist may want to consider double-gloving to protect in the potential event of the outer glove breaking or being cut open on a sharp tooth edge or dental appliance.
- Gloves must be disposed of according to local health department requirements.
- Finger cots if you have a cut finger or open cuticle.

Technical

- Note: Not all of the disease you should be concerned about will be found inside the mouth. In an effort to protect the client and yourself, you need to determine if there are signs of oral:
  - Herpes and/or cold sores
  - Postpone treatment if client is dealing with an active lesion
  - Cuts
  - Burns
- Hand sanitizer (alcohol based) has been shown to provide additional benefit in killing microbes on the hands. Do not use hand sanitizer on gloved hands.
- Be aware that the harshness of some soaps and hand sanitizers can cause the hands to chap and breakout in rashes.
- Immunization should be considered to reduce the possibility of getting disease. You should contact your physician for additional advice. Immunizations may include:
  - Hepatitis B Vaccination
  - Tetanus and Diphtheria
  - Rubella
  - Rubeola (Measles)
  - Mumps
  - Poliomyelitis
  - Tuberculosis
  - Influenza
- Oral rinse, such as Listerine, may be used on the client prior to treatment, to reduce the amount of bacteria present inside the mouth. Oral rinses have been shown to markedly reduce bacterial counts in the mouth. Over the counter rinses can reduce the numbers by 90% for 30-60 minutes after use.
- Surfaces must be decontaminated around the work area.
- All contaminated materials must be disposed of in separate waste bags.

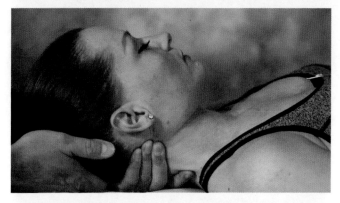

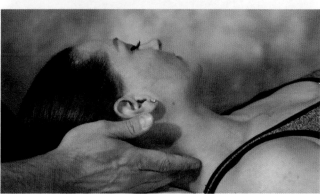

Using hand-over-hand strokes, work briefly to make sure that the tissues are accepting to your work and that your client is comfortable "letting go" of her head and neck. Without saying, "Let go!", encourage the client with statements that relax and help feel the weight of her head. This initial step is not a "warm up" technique, but a fascial "tug", stretching the tissues as you hold and patiently pull along the cervical region into the occiput without lubricants.

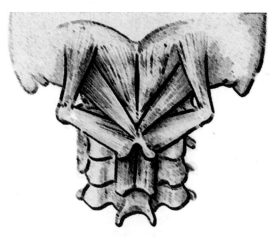

Work trigger points, tender points, spasm and affected areas with specific compressions and cross fiber as needed in the posterior neck. Include the

Superior Trapezius, Splenius Capitis, Splenius Cervicis and Semispinalis Capitis and up into the occiput including the Suboccipital Triangle.

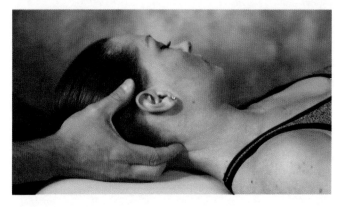

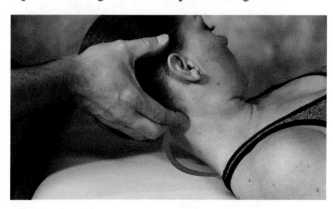

Use pin-and-stretch techniques by lifting the head up and away from the point of pressure. (Analogy: Using the face of a clock as a visual as you sit facing the top of the client's head, her nose is at "noon", her ears are at 9:00pm and 3:00pm and the spinous processes are at 6:00pm. If you are applying pressure to a trigger point at "4:00pm", lift the head and point the client's nose across the clock dial to "10:00pm."

If applying pressure to a trigger point that is at 7:00pm, lift the head and point the client's nose to 1:00pm, etc.

Be sure to use the other hand to support the head and move it away from the pressure for a smooth and consistent stretch. Work within your client's tolerance.

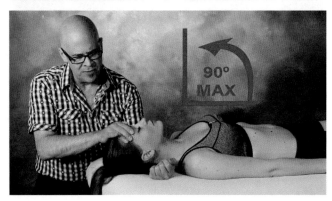

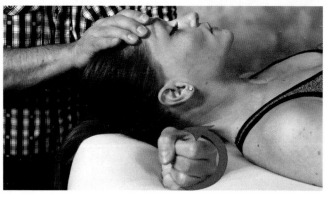

For purposes of decompressing the cervical bones, sit at the head of the table facing your client's head, move to the side of the table that corresponds to your dominant hand (the client's right if you are right-handed and her left side if you are left-handed.) Position yourself at the side of your client's head and place your dominant forearm under your client's neck, using your other hand to lift and support the head as you position yourself.

Firmly applying pressure on your client's forehead with your non-dominant hand, begin by keeping your dominant palm up and gliding your forearm toward her occiput until it is snugly pressing against the occipital ridge. Making a fist with your dominant hand, keeping firm pressure against the occiput,

work at a very slow rate of movement ("slug-like pace") and roll your forearm into internal rotation, applying increasing pressure against your client's occiput. If you are keeping the pressure down on her forehead and your arm pressure against the occiput, you will only be able to turn your forearm up to 90° at most.

Do not allow the pressure to decrease until after you have reached your maximum traction pressure and held it for 15-30 seconds. Begin "unrolling" your tension at the same rate that it was applied until the pressure has completely come off of the occiput.

Note: Suddenly removing the traction can cause extreme spasms in the neck at the atlas/axis.

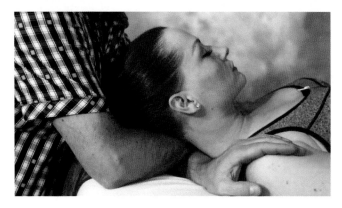

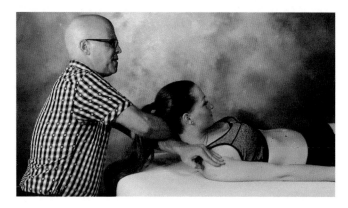

Increasing the anterior neck flexion with PNF, support the head and carefully position your arms so that they are crossed under your client's head, with your hands cupping both of her shoulders at the Deltoid. Starting with your arms resting on the table, your client will push back against your forearms with 20% or so of her strength while she breathes in

deeply for 5-8 seconds. Instruct her to exhale and relax while you gently lift your angle off of the table a couple of inches, stop, hold your position, and have her repeat the resisted extension.

By the end of the 5th cycle, her neck should be almost perpendicular to the table (90 degrees).

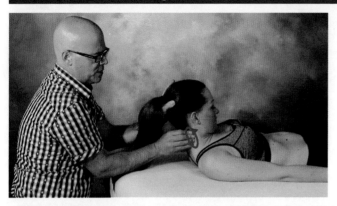

Complete the PNF cervical ROM technique by holding her head at the high-point reached and follow with circular massage on the posterior cervical muscles. No oil. Simply rub the skin over the underlying muscles.

Important Note Before Treating the Anterior Throat and Neck

When working the anterior neck, it is normal to feel a pulse in this area. Pinching or compressing that pulse is not a good idea, however.

There is a mechanism in the carotid artery called the "Carotid Sinus." This mechanism is designed to monitor the body's blood pressure and sudden pressure on the carotid artery, or near it, can sometimes lead the Carotid Sinus to believe the body's blood pressure has suddenly increased. The mechanism reacts by dropping the blood pressure systemically, causing your client to likely pass out. To prevent this, simply ensure any pulse remains next to your fingers, never between them.

Should any technique result in a sharp pain, do not continue the procedure and immediately refer your client to a medical doctor or chiropractor. You should also refer your clients to a chiropractor or medical doctor if the client experiences any dizziness, numbness or tingling sensations.

If you have a client that suffers from a severe headache that has no relief (non-stop, constant) for 3-days or more, do NOT massage the client but immediately recommend the client go to the ER to exclude potential tumor or aneurysm as the source. Massage only when this is excluded as a possibility.

Notes

Migraine (3min heat on neck 1min ice 3min heat) 3X

3 days severe HA does not stop refer them to doctor

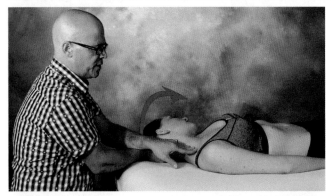

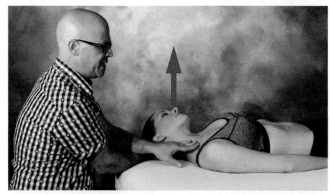

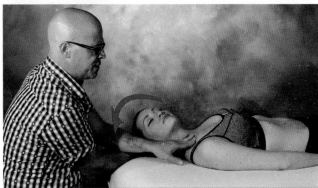

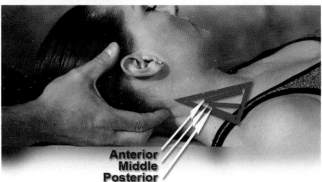

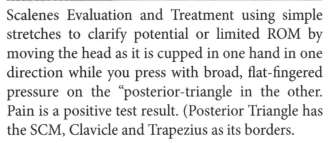

Anterior
Middle
Posterior

Scalenes Evaluation and Treatment using simple stretches to clarify potential or limited ROM by moving the head as it is cupped in one hand in one direction while you press with broad, flat-fingered pressure on the "posterior-triangle in the other. Pain is a positive test result. (Posterior Triangle has the SCM, Clavicle and Trapezius as its borders.

Testing Scalenus Posterior (above left): Client looking left with her left ear to her left shoulder. Press head left while pressing your flat fingers on the posterior area of the Posterior Triangle to the right. Testing Scalenus Medius (above right): Client's left

ear to her left shoulder, her nose towards the ceiling. With flat fingers, press the center of the Posterior Triangle down and to the right as you push her head to the left. To test the Scalenus Anterior, place her head to her left shoulder with her nose pointing right. With flat fingers pressing down and to the right in the anterior part of the Posterior Triangle, press her head to the left.

If pain is present from any of these tests, release the pressure and perform gentle cross-fiber friction and simple, short, gentle "pin & stretch" movements. Go slow and do not over treat.

Client Morning Self-Stretch

It is highly suggested that your client start each day with self-stretches to increase general range of motion and expedite the healing process. Prescribing stretches is not within the scope of practice for all medical professionals so please be aware of your state's laws. Suggesting is usually acceptable, however. Remember on this self stretch to have your client tuck the opposite hand under her buttocks to keep the shoulder from elevating which would decrease the effectiveness of the stretch.

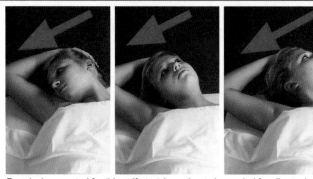

Permission granted for this self-stretch section to be copied for client education.

50

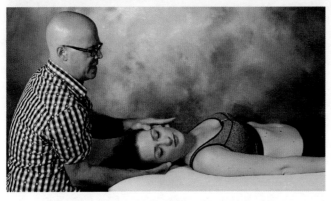

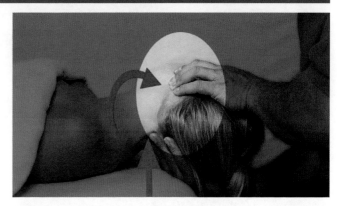

Place your hands on the sides of your client's head, over her ears. Gently turn the head to the right. Your hands should remain mostly parallel. Your right hand's fingers will point toward your client's feet as they support the arch of the neck. Elevate your cli-

ent's head off of the table and draw the SCM from the midpoint of the muscle belly and pin it firmly into the mastoid process. Do not allow your fingers to glide during this technique once they are in place. (Above)

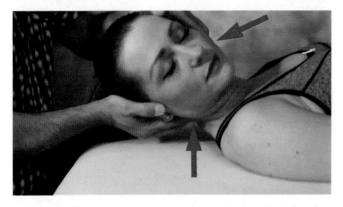

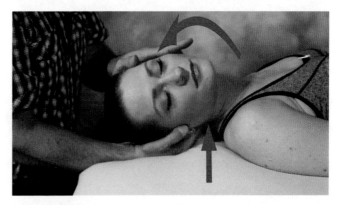

Hold the SCM muscle securely with your left fingertips at the mastoid process of the temporal bone as you drop your client's head back to the table while simultaneously using the length of your fingers of your lower hand to push up against the cervical bones creating a fulcrum (think teeter-totter/see-

saw.) Your hands will parallel each other as you push up. Hold the stretch for about 5-seconds and repeat. Note: You must: 1) maintain firm/non-gliding pressure at the Mastoid Process, 2) push up against the cervical bones. If either is missed, you will lose the stretch.

Notes

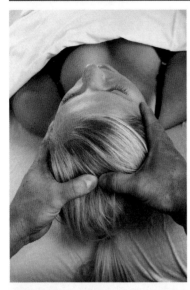

Thumbs pressed down on the crown your client's head as you firmly glide laterally with a slow fascial stretch of the Galea Aponeurotica.

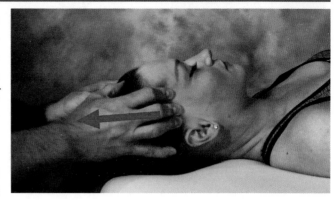

Using your fingers to "rake" through the Temporalis muscle, pulling from just above the Zygomatic Arch (cheek bone), draw slowly and firmly through the tissue until you reach the top of the muscle.

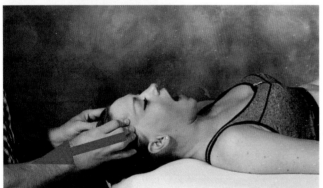

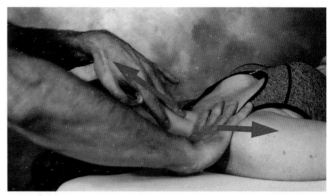

Slowly have your client open her mouth as you drag through the Temporalis muscle for a stretch. Use your broad fingertips to pull apart and stretch the superficial layers and fascia of the Platysma muscle. Work slowly and gently with fascial speed.

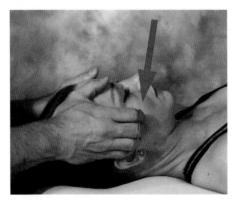

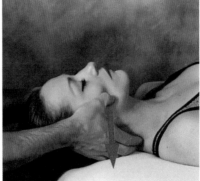

Drag your in-line fingertips just inferior to the Zygomatic Arch, from anterior towards the table. Work deeply and slowly. If the sensation is too intense, work just one side at a time while bracing the head with the other hand. Use your thumbs to "hook" the Masseter, pulling down on it firmly but slowly towards the table. Back the pressure off between 50-75% as you instruct your client to slowly open her jaw for a pin and stretch.

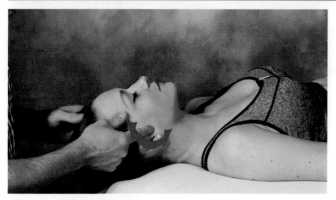
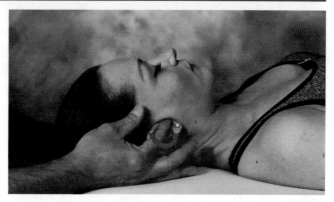

Work methodically around the Temporomandibular Joint, palpating the condyle outside of the ear, anteriorly as well as in the ear via the external acoustic meatus, against the back of the Mandible (Condyle of the Mandible)

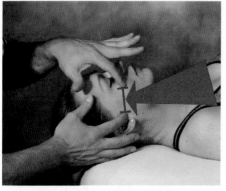
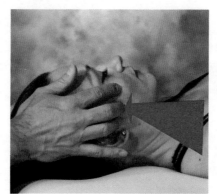
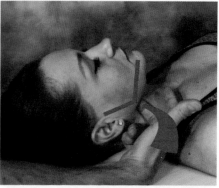

External work on Medial and Lateral Pterygoid Muscles. With firm fingertip pressure, work the lateral Pterygoid muscle (photo below left), just below the lateral Zygomatic Arch. You are working deep to the Masseter, so your pressure will need to be slow, but firm. With a hooked fingertip, work the Medial Pterygoid muscle, just inside the angle of the Mandible. Press firmly, but stay in contact with your client, as it will likely be tender if she is dealing with TMJD issues.

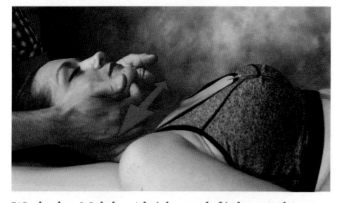
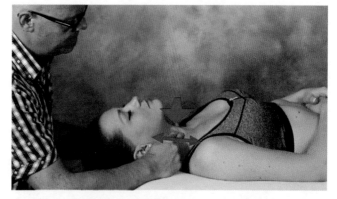

Work the Mylohyoid (above, left) by working to spread and stretch the broad muscle bellies.

Work the Infrahyoid Muscles (Sternohyoid & Sternothyroid) by supporting one side of the Trachea while working along the outer edges on the opposite side using linear friction.

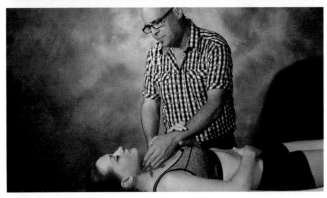

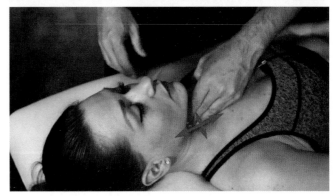

To work the Longus Capitis & Longus Colli, gently displace the trachea from side to side, holding for a moment at the "end feel" (when the trachea will not travel any further laterally.) You can use the length of your thumb to hold the trachea to one side while you drop in with your fingertips on the other side. OR, you can use two fingers on one hand while using two fingers on your other hand, allowing the fingertips to interlace. The interlace is to allow you to work deeply while not displacing a large area of the anterior neck.

Use straight fingertips to palpate and stroke the length of the muscle bellies, followed by cross-fiber friction. You will use the anterior vertebral bodies as a "back board," allowing you to apply pressure on the muscle. This should not feel uncomfortable.

You may need to have your client prop the heel of one foot on the toes of the other foot, and concentrate on balancing the feet to diminish the gag-reflex.

Notes

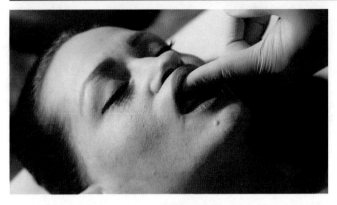

Stretch the fascia on the Maxilla (inside upper lip) by using your fingertip to press up against upper gums with the pad of your finger pressing between lip and upper teeth. Hold pressure and repeat all across from one side to the other.

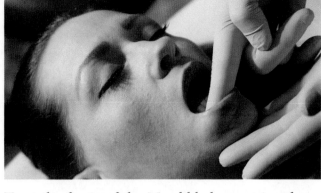

Treat the fascia of the Mandible by pressing down and inward along lower lip against gums. Use the pad of your finger against gums/teeth with the tip of your finger pointing down between lip and gums. Hold and move incrementally all the way across, from side to side.

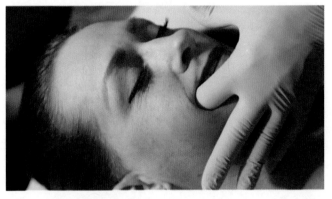

Lateral Pterygoids: Follow the outer edge of the upper molars with your curved finger, gliding upward and inward with finger between Coronoid Process and Teeth, with angle of pressure toward ear. You will be in line with molars up and in as far as possi-

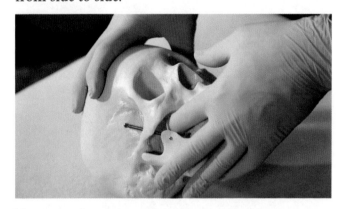

ble upward and inward; work a total of 2-minutes at each spot, applying pressure, making small circles, and occasionally releasing pressure before repeating.

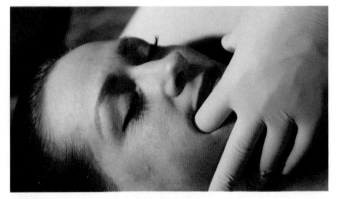

Reach inside cheek, glide towards the TMJ until your finger gets caught in a "U" shaped structure (Sphenomandibular Ligament). Gently press pos-

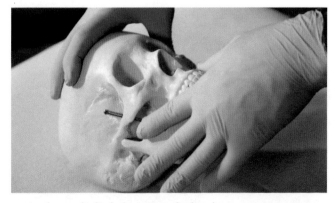

teriorly and slightly toward cheek to get it moving, release fixations and initiate synovial fluid reaction.

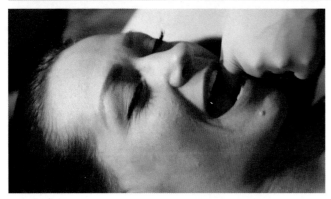

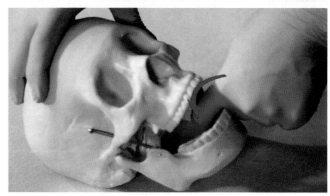

The inferior insertion of the Medial Pterygoids attaches on the Mandible. Slide your finger inside the lower jaw/teeth, along the lower/inside molars. Instruct your client to relax her teeth, resting

them gently on your finger. Once the fingertip is up against the muscle, use the pad of your finger to provide outward pressure.

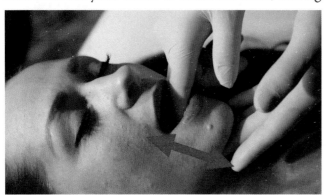

Digastric, Mylohyoid, Geniohyoid, and other muscles on the floor of the mouth can be stretched as you press from outside, below chin and inside mouth. You will feel the pressure of your own fingertips as they come together

Keeping your fingertips together. Slowly stretch the tissues up and down as though you are bouncing on both sides of a trampoline, simultaneously, increasing flexibility of the web of tissues.

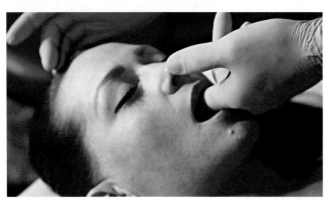

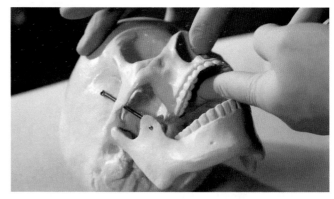

The Palatine Fascia (upper roof of mouth) can be gently stretched with minimal pressure using the pad of your finger, gliding medial to lateral along

dome of the upper palate. Also glide outward and behind back molars.

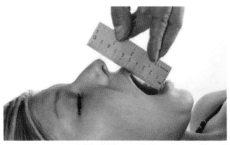

*** Remember to measure the bite opening to determine net change ***

Sequence Reviews

Golfer's Elbow Sequence Review

1. With your client standing, have her hold her arm directly out in front of herself, parallel to the floor with palm to the floor and elbow flexed to 90º. You will be standing in front of her. Press thumb into tender area (distal to medial Epicondyle) and X-fiber friction for 30-seconds.

2. Follow with pressure toward elbow and have the client extend their arm into a straightened position, rolling arm into external rotation, palm ends facing up. Repeat several times

3. Follow with ice.

Tennis Elbow Sequence Review

1. With your client standing, have her hold her or her arm directly out in front of herself, parallel to the floor with palm to the floor and elbow flexed to 90º. Press thumb into tender area (distal to lateral Epicondyle) and X-fiber friction for 30-seconds.

2. Now, stand behind your client and press on the painful area of the tissue with pressure directed toward her Olecranon (elbow point). Pause, and then have the client extend her arm into a straightened position. Repeat several times

3. Follow with ice.

Carpal Tunnel Sequence Review

1. Active/Passive Pin & Stretch of the forearm using shortened-muscle positions

2. Cross-fiber friction the Transverse Ligament and Flexor Retinaculum

3. "Rock & Roll" the wrist, per demonstration

4. Ice the wrist until wrist remains cold for a minute after removing the ice bag

DeQuervain's Sequence Review

1. Perform Finkelstein maneuver to determine appropriateness of technique

2. Gently cross-fiber friction the tendon sheath that is inflamed

3. With your client's hand making a gentle fist, gently Pin & Stretch tendons and tendon sheaths
   - Place hand in fist position
   - Put fist into Radial deviation
   - Apply pressure on tendons and sheath
   - Move fist into ulnar deviation
   - Release and repeat

Seated Sequence Review

1. Palm-glide lateral Trapezius with lateral neck flexion

2. Trapezius pinch with lateral head rotation

3. Pinch posterior cervicals, dropping neck into flexion

4. Lateral Rhomboid glide with torso twist

5. Active/Resistive: Resist your client's attempt to elevate her shoulder while you apply pressure to the Levator Scapula insertion, allowing full range of motion under resistance.

6. Cupped head with circular tips on Suboccipitals and gentle stretch

7. Reinforced fingers/hand (as needed) with pin & stretch all cervical muscle groups (Work around entire neck, 360˚) Rectus Abdominis Treatment

Rectus Abdominus Sequence Review

1. Client supine, legs bent at knee with feet flat on table

2. Client to place their own fingertips at pubic bone for identification of landmark

3. Place your fingers, hand over hand, superior to pubic bone

4. Client takes a deep breath, exhales

5. On exhale, drop down and "under" the pubic bone

6. Hold position while client takes a deep breath for stretch

7. Release and repeat

8. Alternate variation: "Hook" fingertips, with fingers that point straight down towards the table, on the pubic bone, applying cross-fiber friction followed by resisted belly breaths as you hold the lower Rectus Abdominus taut, then release as they exhale.

9. Work upper Rectus Abdominus fibers using parallel thumbs, swinging up and under the lower ribs. Press on the exhale, hold on the inhale with resistance, then release on the next exhale. Repeat 2x on each location, working around the lower ribcage. Use spread thumbs on the center, missing the Xiphoid process.

10. Work from side of table, perpendicular "push & pull" for muscle GTO release

Adductor Sequence Review

1. Client supine; sit at her side. Bend closest leg and place plantar surface of their foot on the table with her toes just under the edge of your thigh.

2. Facing their head, interlock your fingers, making a closed loop with your arms. While the knee is towards the ceiling, apply pressure with inside heel of your hand, pressing on the adductors.

3. Slowly drop knee (external rotation) with pressure on adductors.

4. Release pressure, raise knee and repeat

5. From across the table, use reinforced thumbs and have your client roll her leg into internal rotation, increasing pressure actively on the adductor fibers.

Piriformis Sequence Review

1. Client prone, place flexed leg with flexed knee into external rotation ("Frog-Leg")

2. Static pressure, TP work on sacral border

3. X-Fiber friction at sacral border and Greater Trochanter attachments

4. Bring knees together so they are touching

5. Hold externally rotated leg at the ankle

   • Apply pressure with fist or knuckles at piriformis muscle on sacral border

   • Lift lower leg vertically and toward yourself

   • Release pressure

   • Drop foot toward the other leg

   • Apply pressure and repeat

   • Move upright leg back into external rotation (push away from you.) Use PNF to resist both internal and external rotation of the leg

Gluteus Medius & Minimus Sequence Review

1. Position client on their side at the end of the table, their buttocks flush with the end of the table, knees to chest

2. Work static (TP) pressure on gluteus medius and minimus using "pebble/passive thumb", reinforced thumbs and static elbow.

3. Work with reinforced thumbs up and under Iliac crest, cross-fiber work on Medius/Minimus origins

4. Straighten upper leg with client holding lower leg

5. Passively abduct the leg (lift up); repeat with the client actively lifting their own leg. Using just active motions is preferred.

6. Apply pressure at Gluteus Medius and Minimus with heel of hand [CAUTION: You MUST be certain to keep hips level so that the movement does not laterally flex the low back and potentially damage the client's lumbar facets]

7. Adduct leg toward floor for Pin & Stretch work

IT Band, Knee, Quadriceps, Hamstrings & TFL Sequence Review

SUPINE:

1. Decompress hip with upper thigh drag while client is supine, knee bent, foot is on the table, pull myofascially and lean back.

2. Bend knee, keeping foot on the table, work Medial and Lateral Collateral Ligaments.

3. With lower leg resting on the table without bolster, perform cross-fiber above and below patella using reinforced thumbs.

4. With NO oil, perform a palmar press/myofascial drag from just above knee up leg on at least (3) routes up the thigh.

5. Drop lower leg off table and perform pin & stretch maneuver.

6. Sitting on table edge, drag elbow down groove between "hamstring" muscles using no oil to achieve mechanical and fascial separation.

   - Perform with straight-wristed fist
   - Incorporate "pin & glide" allowing the client to pause and lift actively as you drag.

PRONE:

1. Frog-Leg myofascial "tug" from knee up towards hip.

2. With reinforced thumbs, "strum" across IT Band fibers, broadening them slowly

3. Press down on Sacrum firmly while lifting upper leg with flexed knee slightly off the table - 1" maximum lift. **CAUTION**

4. Bring knees back together: Lift ankle of bent leg and place on your "kneeling thigh" as it rests on the table and slowly press down on her foot, towards her buttocks, stretching the Quadriceps.

SIDE-LYING:

1. Side-lying at edge of table, press your hip into your client's low back. Hold client's knee and ankle as you "wrap" her leg around you, facing away, to stretch her Quads and Psoas.

2. Bring top leg to chest while placing the lower leg in a straight position. Use straight-wristed fist press on medial quads, adductors and hamstrings.

3. TFL: Have client bring knees to chest as they lay as close to the side of the table as possible. Support leg as the flex the hip, medially rotate (ankle up) and abduct the leg (leg raised.)

4. Press on the TFL, holding pressure as they actively extend, eternally rotate and adduct leg.

Sacrum and Pubic Symphysis Release Sequence Review

PRONE:

1. Cross-arm fascial/sacral decompress, working low back and Sacrum, pushing apart

2. X-fiber along sacral borders, Coccyx

3. X-fiber SI Joint

4. On the table top, hovering over client's knees:

   - Bilateral SI joint simultaneous pressure
   - Lift/Press the ASIS/SI joint, alternating pressure, holding 1-2 seconds per side, repeating for 12-repetitions per side

SUPINE:

1. On the table top, hovering over client's bent knees:

   - Between bent knees, press down on both ASIS, towards table
   - Press one ASIS while lifting other PSIS, alternate

2. To release pubic symphysis fixation, use Resisted Adduction/Abduction of knees (knees bent, feet on floor) (ART)

   - From side of table, resist knees trying to separate between my looped arms
   - From side of table, resist knees trying to come together with my crossed arms

Bicipital Tendonitis Sequence Review:

1. Explain the technique to your client, and get verbal consent for discomfort

2. Patient seated or supine

3. Isolate the Bicipital Tendon

4. "Grind" cross-fiber with firm pressure for 30-60 seconds

5. Work with ice cup, directly on the tendon, up and down, "with fiber" for 20 seconds or so.

Supraspinatus Sequence Review:

1. Client seated, arm stabilized behind low back

2. Cross-fiber friction at tendon

3. Ice & Wipe on tendon

Low Back Release Sequence Review:

1. Client prone

2. Stand to client's side, locate lateral edge of the least painful QL

3. Apply pressure with reinforced thumbs or elbow pressure at a 45 degree downward angle

4. Have client flex/extend their pelvis while you hold constant pressure (rise and fall with their movement) for approximately one to two minutes. Repeat on opposite side.

   - When the client is past the acute phase, you can also have them perform a hip-hike, alternate between left/right with elbow pressure as well.

5. Turn client to a supine position

6. Start on the opposite Psoas of her "good" QL

7. Drop in at 45 degree angle at midpoint of lateral torso vs. belly button and between ASIS and lower rib

8. Gently drop deeper with each of 3-4 breath/stretches

9. Verify location of Psoas by having them engage the muscle

10. Hold down pressure, pinning Psoas against Lumbar spine

11. Have client take a deep breath as you hold pressure

12. Release pressure as they exhale and repeat 5-6 times, each side

Shin Splint, Foot & Plantar Fasciitis Sequence Review:

1. Client supine

2. Press foot into table, creating internal rotation and hold: Fist glide on Tibialis Anterior as the client actively plantar-flexes and dorsiflexes her foot

3. Stand at table-side. Reinforced thumbs pointed downward as you apply pressure into Tibialis Anterior at distal end

4. Fully dorsiflex foot and return to full plantar-flexion

5. Release pressure, reposition 1" proximally and repeat until you arrive at most superior origin

6. Work between tendons

7. Pin & stretch tendons as you flex/extend toes as a group

8. Work entire external foot

9. Work around Malleolus

PRONE:

1. Work plantar surface with reinforced thumbs while supporting dorsal surface of the foot with your alternate hand.

2. Use elbow for open-handed "perpendicular to parallel swing"

3. Raise lower leg to vertical position and "palm" the heel as the client's foot rests against your forearm. Use your other hand on your own forearm to stabilize the stretch. Also try calf-grip as you apply pin & stretch.

4. Place foot on your ASIS and use two hands for calf stretches

Pectoralis, back & shoulder Sequence Review:

PRONE:

1. Drag up erectors without oil. Pause to press as you lift your forearm while client breathes into the pressure for TP relief. Use elbow for active release: Resist while client retracts scapulae against elbow pressure.

2. Work posterior cervicals and suboccipitals with compression and local pin & stretch

3. Work "ditch" (lamina groove)

4. Stand at client's side, facing her head, place her arm on her low back

5. Lift and stretch Rhomboid by pulling Scapula away from back (with care and caution)

6. From across table, bring farthest shoulder girdle towards you, then glide Rhomboid fibers as you allow girdle to transition back to the table.

SUPINE:

1. "Local" Pin & Stretch with fingers and thumbs on Pectoralis Minor, spreading/lengthening fascia

2. TP work on Pectoralis Minor belly

3. Pin & Stretch Pectoralis Minor by pressing fist or forearm into Pectoralis Minor as you swing arm overhead ("martial arts block")

Teres Minor & Infraspinatus & Subscapularis (Frozen Shoulder) Sequence Review:

1. With client prone, arm on table, work trigger points along lateral border of the Scapulae

2. Supporting the upper arm, apply pressure on the Teres trigger points as you laterally elevate the client's upper arm along side her head for a pin & stretch.

3. Work trigger points inside Infraspinatus "triangle"

4. Cross-fiber Infraspinatus Tendon at crease of armpit

5. Using extra oil or lotion, lubricate the axillary with sweeping motions until evenly applied

6. Repetitive sweeping motions, dragging your fingertips along table surface, then curve fingertips (locked joints) and lift up as you push the Scapula down with the other hand

7. Press down on the trigger points of the superior belly and inferior belly for up to 10 seconds each, and release

8. Perform "hybrid" PNF techniques with resisted adduction and abduction

Supine Head & Neck Sequence – Review Part 1:

1. Fascial tug as you pull on posterior cervicals (if subacute) NO LOTION OR OIL

2. Specific trigger point and spasm work on posterior cervicals and suboccipitals

3. Suboccipital pin & stretch (pin at occiput and lift up and away from pressure)

4. Forearm roll/traction from side of table

5. Cross-armed PNF/MET

6. Scalenes testing-stretch-release

7. SCM pin & stretch

Supine Head & Neck – Sequence Review Part 2:

1. Occipitofrontalis/Galea Aponeurotica lateral thumb spread

2. Temporalis pin & glide with jaw opening

3. Platysma pull/drag

4. Masseter: fingertip glide

5. Masseter: thumb stretch with jaw opening

6. TMJ: finger around condyles of Mandible (inside and outside of ear area)

7. External work on Medial Pterygoid: Center point below Zygomatic Arch, deep to the Masseter - Press firmly and slowly

8. External work on Lateral Pterygoid: under Ramus/angle of Mandible (hook up and out at angle of Mandible)

9. Spread Mylohyoid with fingertips under chin broadly

10. Infrahyoids: Hold Trachea in place with one hand, massage superficially, superior to inferior along sides of Trachea

11. Stand at side of table: Client balances heel of one foot on toes of the other food while gently grasping your wrist for control. Deviate Trachea several times toward yourself with flat fingers. Hold deviation when your fingers are at the mid-line of chin, drop down until you come to rest on flat surface of anterior neck. Work Longus Capitis/Longus Colli deeply along sides of deviated Trachea.

Intraoral Sequence Review:

1. Fingertip stretch on fascia on Maxilla (inside upper lip)

2. Fingertip stretch on fascia of Mandible (inside lower lip)

3. Lateral Pterygoids (outside upper teeth; hook up and inward)

4. Reach inside cheek, glide towards the TMJ until your finger gets caught in a "U" shaped structure (Sphenomandibular Ligament). Gently press posteriorly and slightly toward cheek to get it moving, release fixations and initiate synovial fluid reaction.

5. Medial Pterygoids (inside lower teeth; hook in and outward, beneath molar roots)

6. Floor of mouth (Digastric, Mylohyoid, Geniohyoid, etc.): Mirrored fingers inside/outside

7. Palatine Fascia (upper, posterior roof of mouth)

Recommended Resources

Videos:

- **Massage with Confidence**, DVD, by Robert B. Haase, LMP, available on Amazon.com
- **Marketing Secrets of a Successful Practice**, DVD set, Haase Myotherapy, available on Amazon.com and Haase Myotherapy

Books:

- **Myofascial Pain and Dysfunction – The Trigger Point Manual Vol. 1 & 2**, Dr. Janet Travell; published by Williams & Wilkins, copyright 1998
- **Anatomy Trains: Myofascial Meridians for Manual and Movement Therapists**, Churchill Livingstone, 2nd edition, 2008

Other:

- Minerals: **Mezotrace** brand minerals. Professional wholesale contact: Becky Hannaford, Lakeside Nutrition, 1-800-662-9966
- Self care tool: **Body Back Buddy**; www.bodyback.com, 800-285-8957
- Foot balm (for cracked heels, extreme odor, etc.): **Khepra Foot Balm**; www.khepra.com, 1-800-367-9799; ask to place a "wholesale" order

After graduating in 1991 from the Brian Utting School of Massage, located in Seattle, WA, Robert Haase, LMP, began a career of research and technique experimentation. Although he received an excellent education at the Brian Utting School, Robert was inquisitive, wanting more. An elective course in cadaver anatomy study at the Bastyr School of Naturopathic Medicine left Robert a bit frustrated at the unnatural state of the tissues being observed.

Two years after graduation, Robert had the opportunity to work at the Thurston County Coroner's office as an autopsy assistant. The experience of performing autopsies alongside pathologists from across Washington State, including the team from Harborview Medical Center, gave him greater insights into actual human anatomy as well as the dynamics of injuries that resulted in death. It was this experience that helped Robert update his own technique and led him to help educate other therapists.

In his early years in the massage profession, Robert was asked to be the Director of Marketing for the National Certification Board for Therapeutic Massage & Bodywork, based on his experience and expertise in business and marketing.

After a decade in the field of massage, Robert started the hospital-based Bodymechanics School of Myotherapy & Massage in the fall of 1999 and began teaching his widely acclaimed Haase Myotherapy® course, *Secrets of Deep Tissue*™, shortly thereafter.

After surviving a devastating surgery in October of 2013 where Robert lost the left half of his tongue due to an aggressive cancer, he completed his radiation and chemotherapy treatments just two months later. Today, Robert is actively creating business and marketing programs, authoring books and traveling for both business and pleasure. He also serves as the Chief Marketing Officer for a Hollywood movie production company, blending his joy of marketing with his love of film.

Robert currently lives in Olympia, Washington and is the proud father of three adult daughters.

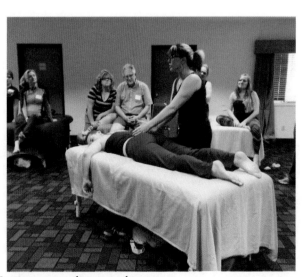

Charity Lisherness, LMP, has been Robert's Assistant Lead Instructor since 2007. Charity is both an instructor as well as on-location seminar manager.

Notes

Made in the USA
Charleston, SC
02 January 2016